7 SHADES OF RED

PERIODS JOURNEY AND MYTHS (CHUMMING)

HANISHA VARMA

Contents

Preface

Periods... Every month blood releases from the women body for 5 days and for some women it even takes more than 7 days.........

Let's talk about Period Struggles every girl / woman can related to!

Menstruation demands careful attention to hygiene to ward off infections and uphold well-being. Historically, women predominantly used cloth to manage menstrual hygiene. Yet, as time progressed, various approaches have surfaced to uphold cleanliness and diminish health risks. Some contend that these customs stemmed from concerns regarding contamination and hygiene, while others propose they were aimed at affording women respite, sparing them from tasks like pickle making, which held considerable significance in numerous households during that era.

"I plan to share various anecdotes and myths related to menstruation, some of which are based on personal experiences of mine or my friends, while others stem from friends and sisters' experiences encounters during their menstrual cycles.

With this book I feel so grateful that I am able to express myself, I am able to communicate to the world right here, right now, and with this i have initiated step to talk about menstruation and its experience openly.

As an ***author***, I hope to share what I've learned from my own body during menstruation, along with the experiences of my sisters and friends, to help guide young girls as they approach their first period. By reflecting on the mistakes made and offering the right methods to prevent them, my aim is to help them embrace this new phase with confidence and positivity. If you're willing to be a student of life, the opportunities for growth are limitless."

1
The Arrival

Tummy hurts when you get your period body is squeezing uterus like lemon, kind of juicing it, so you get pain, because of squeezing you get cramps, you are not able to do your daily stuff, so many girls take a Pill and try to Chill. I also take two medicines on my monthly arrival one is to reduce pain so I can do my daily stuff with little fake smile on my face and I don't puke wherever standing and doing my daily stuff. Funny noooooooooso.

After 18 years of periods, it sounds so funny (for my self). During period arrival mostly on first day tummy makes a girl cry and her tummy is telling her to sleep otherwise I will kick you so hard so you will remove water from mouth along with uterus.

Arrival Feeling experience

There's nothing quite like the suspense of waiting for your period to arrive. It's a bit like waiting for a package you didn't order, but you know it's coming anyway. And not just any package—one that might explode on arrival, ruining everything in its vicinity.

Every trip to the bathroom becomes a suspenseful event. You're like a detective, inspecting the evidence to see if today's the day. But nope, it's just a false alarm. The disappointment (or is it relief?) mix depend on every month my schedule.

You start questioning your body's sense of timing. Why can't it just stick to the schedule? Isn't it supposed to be like clockwork?

?

It's that time of the month again. You're going about your day, feeling fine, and then suddenly, everything feels different. You start feeling a little more irritable, the smallest things annoy you, and you wonder why your emotions are running high. You snap at your siblings, your friends, or even your favorite show. Deep down, you know something's up.

For many of us, these mood swings aren't random—they're a clear sign that our period is about to arrive. It's as if our body is sending out signals to prepare us. Along with these emotional shifts, you might notice something else: a bit of white discharge. This discharge, which can be normal for many women, is often a prelude to your period, like your body's way of saying, "Get ready, it's coming soon."

As the days progress, some mild cramping might begin in your lower abdomen. It's not the full-on period pain yet, but a gentle reminder that things are about to start. You might also feel bloated, like your stomach is tighter than usual, or even experience a bit of constipation. It's frustrating, especially when you're trying to go about your daily routine.

Flashback..............

I remember one day when I was about 15. I woke up with a slight tummy ache and just felt off all day. Every little thing set me off, and my mood was all over the place. Later that evening, I noticed some discharge in my body. I knew something change in my body but I was scared and was making crying face in front of my mom so she can pamper me and take care of me. I asked my mum about incident of giving pads in my school and I asked her what is it, when I was in my 16 my mum was bit hesitate to talk anything on periods openly so my mom just cut the topic and said when time will come will tell u, I started crying holding my stomach and she got doubt she has taken me to washroom and checked me and declared that u got ur periods and started explaining me the process, cycle, why and all. While it was a relief to finally know what was happening, those days leading up to it were always a rollercoaster of emotions and physical discomfort.

Breaking the Silence: How to Approach Period Conversations

It's a powerful moment when a girl first experiences her period, and it's crucial for both mothers and daughters to handle it with care and openness.
If a girl feels hesitant to talk about her period with her own mother, it's important to remember that she is not alone. Many girls, especially in cultures where menstruation isn't openly discussed, find it hard to initiate this conversation. Here are a few gentle steps a girl can take if she's unsure how to approach her mother:

1. **Choose a Comfortable Moment**: Look for a relaxed time, like during a meal or a casual outing, when both you and your mom aren't distracted or rushed. This creates a safe space for a private and important talk.

2. **Ask Simple, Direct Questions**: You don't have to dive straight into the deep details. Start by asking your mom about her own experience. "Mom, I remember you mentioning something about periods. Can you tell me more?" This will help ease the conversation without overwhelming either of you.

3. **Use a Story or Example**: If it's still tough to bring it up directly, talk about a friend's experience or something you read online, "I was reading about periods, and it made me think—what should I expect?" This can open the door to more detailed discussions.

How Mothers Can Create a Supportive Environment

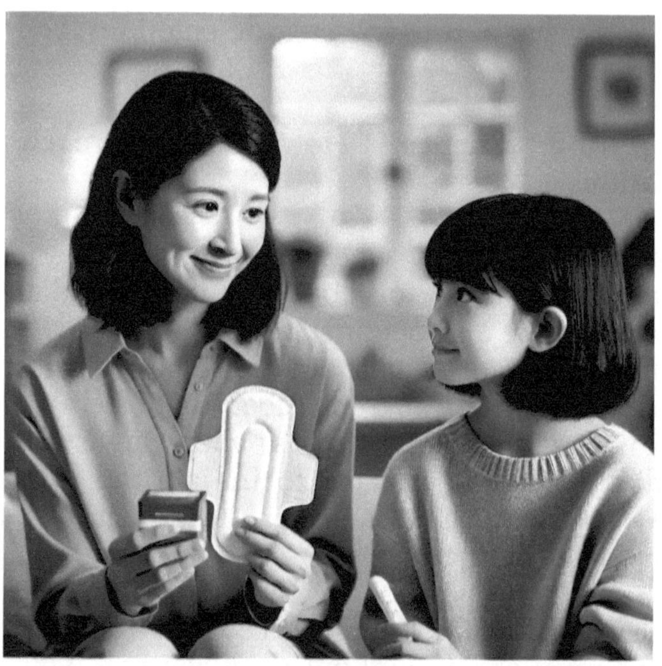

For mothers, this is a precious opportunity to create a bond based on trust, understanding, and support. When your daughter begins asking about periods, it's important to handle it with openness and sensitivity. Here's how:

1. **Be Open and Honest**: Even if you feel hesitant, remember your daughter is coming to you for guidance. Answer her questions honestly, using simple language, and avoid making the topic feel taboo or uncomfortable.

2. **Acknowledge Her Feelings**: Your daughter might feel scared, confused, or embarrassed. Acknowledge these emotions and reassure her that it's completely normal to feel this way. Let her know that you understand and that you went through the same process.

3. **Create a Calm and Reassuring Atmosphere**: A calm tone can make all the difference. If your daughter feels emotional or confused, comfort her with a hug or sit next to her while explaining the process gently. The goal is to make her feel safe and cared for.

4. **Provide Simple, Clear Information**: Explain the basics of menstruation, the cycle, and what she can expect physically and emotionally. Use real-life examples or even books and videos that might help her understand better. Avoid making it sound too scientific or scary.

5. **Encourage Ongoing Conversations**: One talk won't cover everything. Let your daughter know she can come to you with any questions or concerns in the future, even if they seem embarrassing or difficult. This creates a foundation of trust for other conversations down the line.

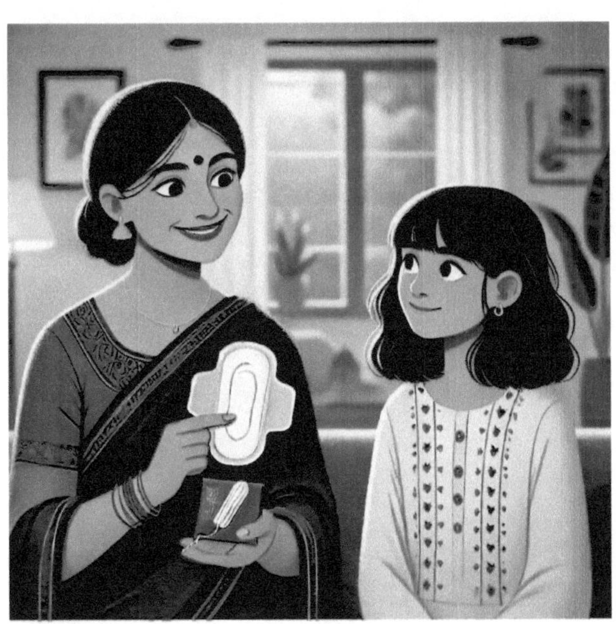

The first period is an important rite of passage, and handling it with sensitivity, care, and open dialogue helps make the experience less daunting and more empowering for both the girl and her mother. If you find it hard to talk about periods, know that this moment can be a beautiful opportunity for understanding and growth between you and your mom.

2

Kash Ye periods Advertising Jese easy hote

"If Only Periods Were as Easy as Advertised..."

Imagine a world where periods are just like in the advertisements: a gentle breeze blows through your hair as you effortlessly jog down the beach, smiling, because you're wearing the latest ultra-absorbent pad that promises to keep you dry and comfortable for 12 hours straight. The reality, as we all know, is far less glamorous.

Let's take a trip into the world of period commercials, where everything seems perfect. You wake up refreshed, no cramps in sight, and of course, your pad is like a soft, fluffy cloud that keeps you dry even during an intense workout. "Ha!" we laugh in unison.

In reality, waking up on the first day of your period is more like being hit by a truck. Your lower abdomen feels like it's been twisted into a knot, you're bloated enough to float like a balloon, and there's a small army of pimples staging a coup on your face. But of course, the pad you put on last night somehow managed to shift, leaving you with that delightful sensation of dampness where you least want it.

Let's talk about those super active, always-smiling women in the ads who can do anything during their periods. They swim, they run, they do yoga, all while grinning like they just won the lottery. Meanwhile, the rest of us are curled up in the fatal position on the couch, clutching a hot water bottle and binging on chocolate like our lives depend on it.

And the catchphrases! "Feel confident all day long," they say. Sure, because nothing screams confidence like the constant fear of leaking through your clothes in the middle of a meeting. Or better yet, the awkward shuffle to the bathroom with your pad or tampon hidden in your sleeve, because despite it being 2024, we're still doing the secret-agent move with our period supplies.

One of the most unrealistic expectations these commercials set is the idea that periods can be completely hidden. You know the type: the pad is so thin, it's basically invisible! You can wear those skin-tight white pants with no worries. Newsflash: nobody with a shred of sanity wears white pants during their period. In fact, many of us have a special wardrobe reserved for that time of the month—loose, dark, and preferably stretchy.

But let's not forget the tampons. The ads would have us believe that inserting a tampon is as easy as popping a Tic Tac into your mouth. In reality, it's more like trying to thread a needle while blindfolded and upside down. And then there's the anxiety that comes with wondering if you've inserted it correctly, if it's going to leak, or if you're about to become the next victim of toxic shock syndrome.

There's also the magical "overnight protection" myth. According to ads, you can sleep like a baby without worrying about leaks. But anyone who's experienced the dreaded "crime scene" upon waking knows that the reality is far messier. You end up sleeping in a position so awkward, it could be mistaken for advanced yoga, all in an attempt to keep everything in place.

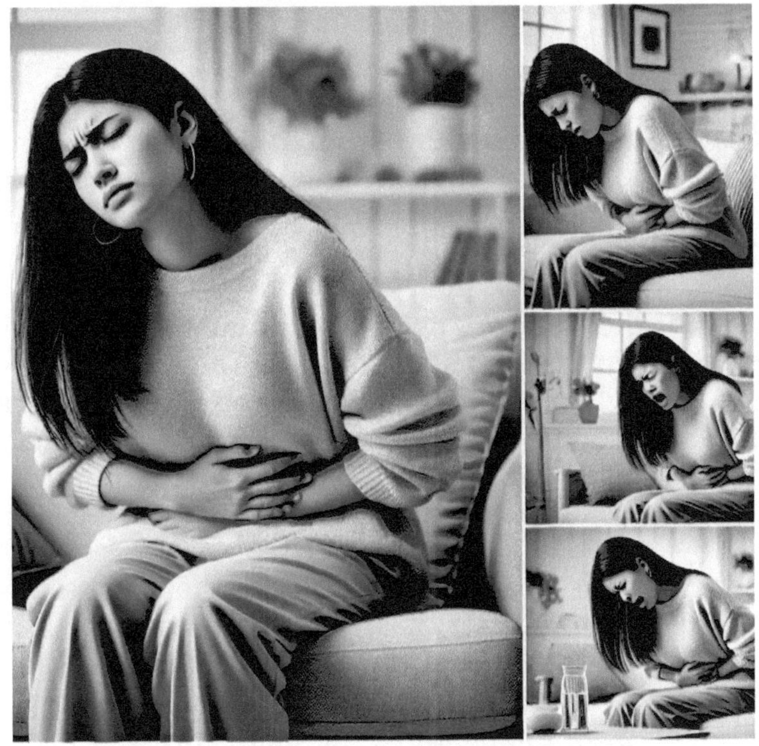

Actual Feeling before and during periods

There's the constant battle with your wardrobe. You carefully select clothes that are both comfortable and capable of concealing any potential accidents. Dark colors are your best friends, while white pants are your sworn enemies. You feel like a soldier preparing for battle, except your armor is a pair of granny panties and your weapon of choice is a super-absorbent pad.

The paranoia doesn't stop there. Every slight cramp or mood swing has you on high alert. "Is this it? Is this the beginning?" you ask yourself as you reach for the chocolate that you swore you wouldn't touch. Suddenly, you're not sure if you're bloated or if you've just eaten an entire family-sized bag of chips in one sitting.

And let's not forget the emotional rollercoaster. One minute, you're perfectly fine, and the next, you're tearing up at a commercial about paper towels. Is it PMS, or are you just losing it? Who knows? You certainly don't. But you do know that you're a ticking time bomb of emotions, ready to burst into tears or laughter at the drop of a hat.

Then comes the phantom period symptoms. You're convinced it's starting. You feel the cramps, the bloating, the whole shebang. But when you check, there's nothing. Your period is playing an elaborate game of hide and seek, and you're losing. It's like that annoying friend who says they're "on their way" but shows up two hours late.

Just when you've resigned yourself to the idea that your period is going to be late, it arrives. And not with a gentle knock, but with a full-blown, door-kicking entrance. Suddenly, all those symptoms you were dreading come rushing in at once. The cramps, the bloating, the mood swings—they're all here, and they've brought friends.

Your period's arrival is never at a convenient time. It's as if it has a personal vendetta against you. It shows up when you're in the middle of a meeting, or worse, when you're out and about with no supplies in sight. Cue the panic as you frantically search for a pad or tampon, mentally cursing your period for its terrible timing.

And then there's the "welcome party" you have to throw for yourself. You know the drill: hot water bottle, comfy pants, and a stockpile of snacks that could feed a small army. You curl up in bed, ready to ride out the storm, only to realize that your period is just getting started. It's going to be a long few day.

But despite all the stress, the paranoia, and the inevitable mess, there's a weird sense of relief when your period finally arrives. It's like the suspense is over, and now you can just deal with it. Sure, it's inconvenient and uncomfortable, but at least the waiting game is over.

So, you settle into your routine, knowing that in a few days, this will all be behind you—until next month, when the whole cycle starts again. But for now, you've got this. You're ready to handle whatever your period throws at you, with a sense of humor and maybe a few extra pieces of chocolate.

In conclusion, if periods were anything like the advertisements, we'd all be living in a no place of perfectly balanced hormones, stain-free sheets, and unlimited energy. But they're not. And that's okay. Because we, the real women, know that periods are messy, uncomfortable, and sometimes downright painful. But they're also a part of life. And if we can't laugh at the absurdity of it all, what can we do?

So here's to embracing the chaos, the bloating, the cramps, and yes, even the occasional leak. Because while periods might not be as easy as the ads suggest, they're a lot easier to handle when we face them with a sense of humor and a healthy dose of reality.

3

U Get Ur Period When U Plan for FUN

"Murphy's Law of Periods: Fun Plans Equal Period Arrival"

There's a universal truth that every woman knows: periods have the worst timing. It's almost like they have a built-in radar for when you've planned something fun, exciting, or important, and they decide, "Yup, this is the perfect time to show up!" Whether it's a vacation, a big date, or even a once-in-a-lifetime event, you can almost guarantee that your period will crash the party.

Let's start with vacations. You've been planning for weeks, maybe even months. You've packed the perfect swimsuit, bought new sundresses, and stocked up on sunscreen. You're ready for the ultimate relaxation—sun, sand, and sea. And then, the night before you leave, you feel it. **CRAMP.** "No, please, not now," you plead with your body. But your uterus has other plans. You wake up the next morning to find that Aunt Flo has decided to join you on your trip.

So instead of lounging by the pool, you're dealing with cramps, and the constant worry of leaking through your bikini. You're forced to swap out that white swimsuit for something darker, and your relaxing days in the sun are now punctuated by frequent bathroom trips and the discreet disposal of pads or tampons. And forget about the beach volleyball game you were so excited for—jumping and running are the last things you want to do right now.

Then there's the issue of food. You were looking forward to indulging in delicious vacation treats, but instead, your period has triggered cravings so intense that you end up eating everything in sight. And not in a cute, "I'm on vacation, I deserve this" way, but in a "give me all the chocolate or I'll cry" kind of way. You're halfway through a decadent dessert when you realize that you've just single-handedly consumed enough calories to fuel a marathon, but hey, who's counting?

And let's not forget about romantic getaways. You've planned the perfect weekend with your partner—a cozy cabin in the woods, a bottle of wine, and no distractions. Everything is set for a weekend of romance. But as you're packing your bags, you feel that familiar twinge in your lower abdomen. "No, not this weekend!" you silently scream. But it's too late. Your period has decided to make it a trio.

Now, instead of romantic nights by the fire, you're dealing with cramps that feel like a medieval torture device is at work inside your body. The lingerie you bought? Forget about it. You're in full comfort mode—sweatpants, oversized T-shirt, and a hot water bottle permanently glued to your belly. And while your partner is understanding, you can't help but feel a little cheated out of the weekend you had planned.

It's not just vacations or romantic getaways either. Your period seems to have a knack for showing up at every major life event. Got a wedding to attend? Great! Time to find a dress that's both stylish and capable of concealing any potential mishaps. But of course, you end up spending most of the reception worrying about whether your pad is still in place and whether anyone can tell you're wearing what feels like a diaper underneath your fancy attire.

Or how about that big presentation at work? You've been

prepping for weeks, and now it's your time to shine. But as you're about to step up to the podium, you feel that unmistakable gush. Suddenly, your focus shifts from delivering a killer presentation to ensuring that you don't have a wardrobe malfunction in front of your colleagues. You're giving your speech with one part of your brain on autopilot, while the other part is desperately calculating how much longer you have until you can safely retreat to the bathroom.

Even birthdays aren't safe. You've planned a night out with friends, you're wearing your best outfit, and you're ready to celebrate. But guess who decides to make an appearance? That's right—your period. Now you're dealing with cramps, mood swings, and the general annoyance of having to excuse yourself to the bathroom every hour. The worst part? Your friends have surprised you with a cake and a round of shots, and all you can think about is how much you'd rather be in bed with a heating pad.

So I have multiple memories of my periods arrived on wrong time but wanna share latest one and memorable one.

Surprise! It's That Time Again – and at Mrs. India competition, No Less!

So, picture this: I'm all set to participate in the Mrs. India pageant in 2023, feeling fabulous, confident, and, of course, with my period a solid *eight days* away. It had been so predictable over the past six months, I didn't even give it a second thought. But, as the universe would have it, nerves + global stage = surprise early period! Yep, it decided to show up uninvited—*the night before* the big event.

Cue: panic mode. I usually pop two trusty pills a day to keep my sanity in check, but guess what? It's 5 AM, I'm in Delhi, unfamiliar with the area, and I'm frantically hunting for a medical shop like I'm on some sort of scavenger hunt—except the prize is pain relief. And, oh, just to add a sprinkle of chaos, I'm surrounded by drop-dead gorgeous women while stress is skyrocketing about how to look like a queen while feeling like a *disaster*.

But here's the thing about being a woman—when life throws us a curveball like this, somehow, we get a little boost from the universe, a *divine superpower* that helps us rise to the occasion. And guess what? I did. I survived (thank you, medicine gods!) and even snapped a few nervous selfies right after changing into my outfit. Oh, the thoughts that were racing through my head: "How on earth am I going to strut in 6-inch heels, bleeding, and still look like a

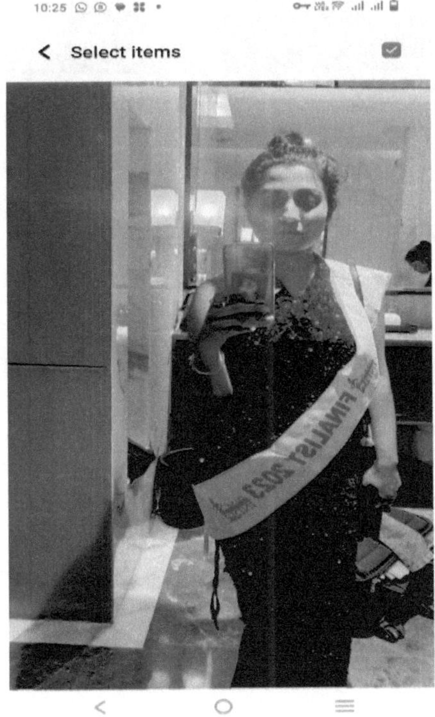

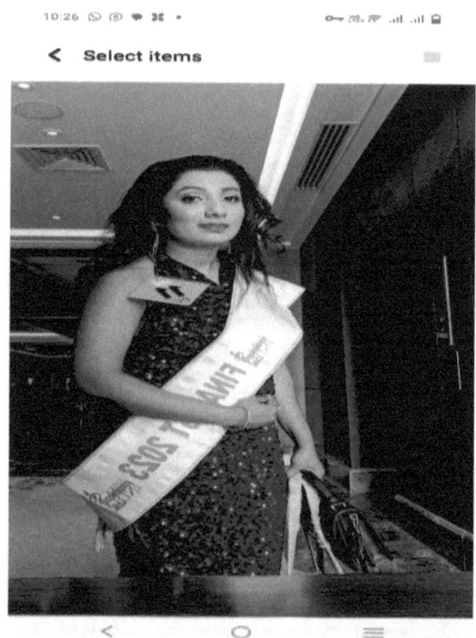

Spoiler alert: I survived. And not only did I survive—I *thrived*. I went on to win the title of Mrs. Maharashtra! But let me tell you, those first three days of the event, with practice sessions on heels and everything, were a whole different level of challenging. Blood, sweat, and heels—literally!

But here's the thing—despite its terrible timing, you learn to roll with it. You pack extra supplies, choose your outfits wisely, and keep a sense of humor about the whole situation. Because as frustrating as it is to have your period crash every fun event, it's not going to stop you from enjoying life. You find ways to adapt, whether it's packing a discreet period kit for vacations or having a backup plan for those big events.

And sometimes, you just have to laugh. Because if you didn't, you'd cry, and then you'd probably blame it on the hormones. So here's to making the best of it, to dancing at weddings in your black dress, to rocking that bikini with confidence, and to giving that presentation like the boss you are, even if you're fighting a battle with your own body.

Because periods may have the worst timing, but you've got the best attitude. And that's what makes all the difference.

4

Facts About Women's Bodies

"The Truth About Women's Bodies: A Hilarious Guide to the Crazy, Wonderful, and Bizarre"

Let's be honest—women's bodies are nothing short of miraculous. They can create life, endure mind-boggling pain, and bounce back from almost anything. But they're also full of quirks, mysteries, and downright bizarre facts that make you wonder if Mother Nature was having a bit of fun when she designed us. So, let's dive into some of the wildest, most fascinating facts about women's bodies, served up with a healthy dose of humor.

Fact #1: Women are born with all the eggs they'll ever have. That's right, ladies—before you were even born, you were packing heat. By the time you were born, your ovaries were already stocked with about one to two million eggs. It's like being born with a lifetime supply of lottery tickets, except instead of winning money, you get periods and the potential for pregnancy. But here's the kicker: by the time you hit puberty, half of those eggs have already given up and gone home. So really, it's like a rigged lottery where most of your tickets are duds.

Fact #2: The menstrual cycle is technically a monthly rehearsal for pregnancy. Every month, your body gets all dressed up with nowhere to go. It's like your uterus throws a party, gets everything ready, and then—just when it's time for the guests to arrive—realizes it sent out the wrong invitations. So, what happens? The decorations get torn down, the snacks are thrown away, and the party is canceled until next month. And by "decorations," we mean the uterine lining, and by "torn down," we mean, well, you know the drill.

Fact #3: Women have a higher pain threshold than men. Sorry, guys, but it's true. Studies have shown that women can tolerate more pain than men—probably because we have to deal with periods, childbirth, and high heels. But just because we can handle it doesn't mean we enjoy it. Remember that the next time you see a woman smiling through the pain of cramps or the agony of waxing. It's not that it doesn't hurt—it's just that we're too stubborn to let it show.

Fact #4: Women's brains are wired for multitasking. You've probably heard the joke that women can do multiple things at once while men can only focus on one thing at a time. Well, there's some truth to that. Research suggests that women's brains are better equipped for multitasking, which is why we can hold a conversation, cook dinner, and mentally plan tomorrow's outfit all at the same time. Of course, this also means that our brains are constantly juggling a million things, which might explain why we sometimes forget where we put our keys. Which is why sometimes we get confuse in performing task. But there is no choice even corporate woman who is CEO of firm has to decide the meal and tell her cook what needs to be prepared.

Fact #5: The uterus is a seriously strong muscle. The uterus isn't just for show—it's one of the strongest muscles in the human body. It has to be, considering it's responsible for pushing a human being out during childbirth. That's right—the same organ that causes you so much grief every month is also capable of the Herculean task of labor. And when it's not busy being a powerhouse, it's working hard to shed its lining every month like a loyal (if somewhat overzealous) cleaning crew.

Fact #6: Women's skin is thinner than men's. Ever wonder why women's skin tends to be softer, but also more prone to wrinkles? It's because our skin is thinner than men's, which makes it more delicate and, unfortunately, more susceptible to the effects of aging. On the bright side, this also means we have an excuse to splurge on all those fancy skincare products. After all, we're just protecting our delicate epidermis, right?

Fact #7: Women's immune systems are stronger than men's. Here's something to cheer about: women tend to have stronger immune systems than men. That's why we're less likely to get sick, and when we do, we often recover faster. Scientists think this might be because women have to protect their bodies—and any potential pregnancies—from all sorts of invaders. So next time the flu is going around, you can thank your supercharged immune system for keeping you healthy.

Fact #8: Women's sense of smell is more sensitive. Women generally have a better sense of smell than men, which is both a blessing and a curse. On the one hand, it means we can enjoy the subtle nuances of a fine perfume or detect the aroma of freshly baked cookies from a mile away. On the other hand, it also means we're more likely to be overwhelmed by bad smells—like that mysterious odor coming from the fridge that no one else seems to notice.

Fact #9: Women's bodies are designed for endurance. When it comes to physical endurance, women have the edge. We're built to go the distance, which is probably why we can power through long hours of work, take care of the family, and still have enough energy to binge-watch our favorite shows at the end of the day. It's also why women excel in endurance sports like marathons and long-distance swimming. So next time you're feeling worn out, just remember—you're built for this.

Fact #10: Women are natural nurturers—thanks to oxytocin.
Oxytocin, often called the "love hormone," plays a big role in
bonding and nurturing behavior. It's why women are so good
at caring for others, whether it's comforting a friend, taking
care of a child, or even just listening to someone's problems.
But oxytocin isn't all warm and fuzzy—it's also the hormone
that helps trigger labor contractions. So, while it makes us feel
all lovey-dovey, it's also responsible for some serious pain.

So there you have it—some of the most fascinating (and
funny) facts about women's bodies. We're strong, resilient,
and yes, a little bit weird, but that's what makes us awesome.
Our bodies may be complex, but they're also incredibly
capable. So next time you're feeling frustrated with your body,
just remember how amazing it truly is. And maybe laugh
a little, too—because if we can't laugh at the strange and
wonderful things our bodies do, then what's the point?

One moment you're laughing at a silly joke, and the next,
you're overwhelmed with tears, wondering why everything
feels so intense—mood swings during your period can be like
riding an emotional imbalance. But while we can't always
control the ups and downs, we *can* find ways to keep our
bodies calm and centred through the storm.

1. **Managing Mood Swings**: Mood swings before your period
   are a result of fluctuating hormones, particularly estrogen
   and progesterone. To manage these, it's essential to prioritize
   self-care during this time. Here are a few tips:

   - **Stay Active**: Light exercise like walking or yoga can release
     endorphins, which naturally improve your mood.
   - **Relaxation Techniques**: Deep breathing, meditation, or
     even spending time in nature can help calm those
     heightened emotions.
   - **Healthy Diet**: Try to avoid too much caffeine or sugar,
     as they can make mood swings worse. Instead, focus on
     balanced meals with lots of fruits, vegetables, and whole

grains.

2. **Handling Tummy Pain and Bloating:** A slight tummy ache before your period is common and usually mild compared to the cramps that can come later. However, it can still be uncomfortable:

   - **Heat Therapy:** Applying a warm water bottle or heating pad to your lower abdomen can relax the muscles and ease discomfort.
   - **Stay Hydrated:** Drink plenty of water to help reduce bloating. Avoid salty foods, as they can make bloating worse.
   - **Ginger or Chamomile Tea:** These can soothe your digestive system and help with both cramping and constipation.

3. **Dealing with Constipation:** Hormonal changes can slow down your digestive system, leading to constipation. To keep things moving:

   - **Increase Fiber:** Add more fruits, vegetables, and whole grains to your diet. Foods like apples, prunes, and oats are particularly good.
   - **Stay Hydrated:** Drinking enough water is key in preventing constipation.
   - **Move Around:** Physical activity can help stimulate digestion and prevent constipation.

4. **Understanding White Discharge:** White discharge before your period is usually normal and a sign that your period is coming soon. However, it's essential to recognize what's typical for your body:

   - **Keep Clean:** Wear cotton underwear and change them regularly to stay fresh.
   - **Track Your Cycle:** By tracking your discharge and other symptoms, you can predict when your period is about to

start and be better prepared.

In the end, the key is to listen to your body. Everyone's experience is unique, but by tuning into the signals, you can prepare yourself both physically and mentally for your period's arrival. These changes might feel inconvenient, but they're your body's way of keeping things in balance. And with the right approach, you can minimize the discomfort and even find some peace in the process.

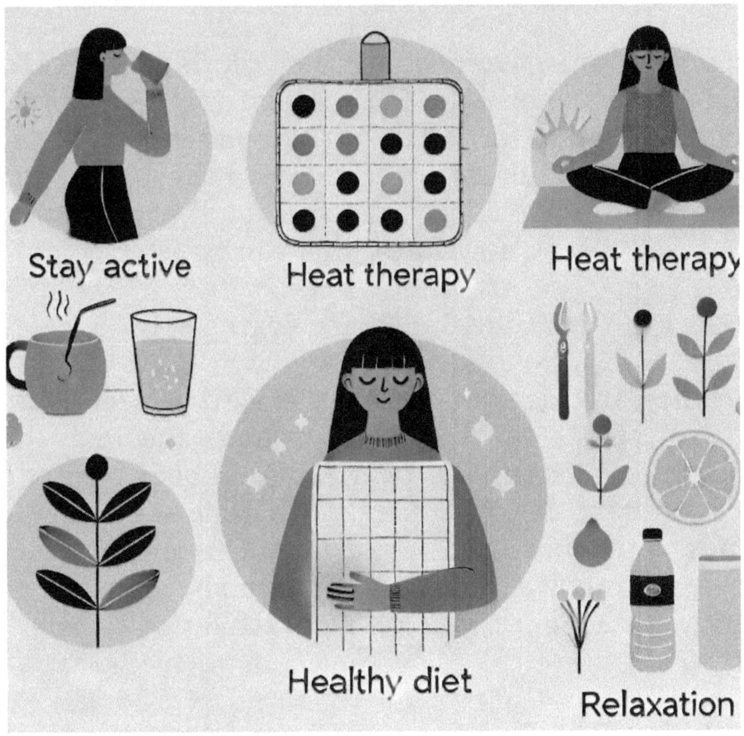

Understanding Sugar Response Changes During the Menstrual Cycle

Ever wondered why your body's reaction to sugar seems to change throughout your menstrual cycle? The reason lies in the delicate interplay of hormones that regulate your cycle and affect how your body processes and utilizes sugar. No two weeks are the same, and here's why.

The menstrual cycle's primary purpose is to prepare for potential pregnancy by growing and releasing an egg from the ovaries. This process is divided into four main phases:
    1. **Follicular Phase (Days 1-13)**
    2. **Ovulation (Days 14-15)**
    3. **Luteal Phase (Days 16-28)**
    4. **Menstrual Phase (End of Cycle)**

These phases are governed by four key hormones: Follicle-Stimulating Hormone (FSH), Luteinizing Hormone (LH), Estrogen (Estradiol or E2), and Progesterone (PG). These hormones also influence how your body responds to sugar, affecting insulin sensitivity, glucose uptake, and even your cravings. Let's break down how this works:

Week 1: The Follicular Phase Begins

During the early days of your cycle, estrogen levels are low while FSH begins to rise, which signals the body to start developing follicles in the ovaries. Your body's response to sugar is quite balanced during this phase—neither overly insulin-sensitive nor insulin-resistant. This means that sugar cravings are relatively low, and your body manages glucose efficiently, as long as you don't overindulge in high-sugar foods.

Week 2: The Proliferative Phase – Embrace the Sweet Treats

As you enter the second week, estrogen levels rise steadily, making your body more insulin-sensitive. When your body becomes more insulin-sensitive, your muscle cells are better able to absorb glucose from the bloodstream, making this the ideal week to enjoy a little indulgence with sugary foods and desserts. Your body can handle the extra glucose without causing major spikes or storing it as fat.

Ovulation: Hormonal Highs and Changing Responses

Around the middle of your cycle, estrogen peaks, and LH surges to trigger ovulation. This hormonal shift makes you feel more energetic and euphoric but also temporarily increases insulin resistance. This means that your body may not process sugar as efficiently as it did in Week 2, leading to slight fluctuations in blood sugar levels. During this phase, it's best to keep simple sugar intake moderate to avoid any unnecessary spikes.

Week 3: The Luteal Phase – The Sugar Rollercoaster

After ovulation, the luteal phase begins, and progesterone levels rise significantly. This hormone induces insulin resistance, meaning your body struggles to efficiently utilize glucose, which can lead to higher sugar levels in the bloodstream. This is why you might crave more sugary or carb-heavy foods during this week. However, be cautious: indulging these cravings can cause your body to store excess glucose as fat, leading to fatigue and weight gain. The best approach is to focus on complex carbs and maintain steady blood sugar levels.

Week 4: Menstrual Phase or Early Pregnancy Changes

If fertilization does not occur, progesterone levels start to drop during Week 4, bringing your insulin sensitivity back to normal. You might notice that your sugar cravings and energy levels become more stable. If fertilization does occur, progesterone continues to rise, and the body remains in a state of insulin resistance to store glucose for future energy needs. In this case, it's important to avoid refined sugars to prevent heightened insulin resistance and further cravings.

Final Thoughts: Listen to Your Body

Understanding how your body's response to sugar changes during each phase of your cycle can empower you to make informed dietary choices. The most optimal time to enjoy sugary foods is during Week 2, when your body is most insulin-sensitive, while Week 3 is the trickiest, as it's more likely to cause blood sugar fluctuations and weight gain. Awareness and planning can help you maintain your energy, reduce fatigue, and better manage your overall health throughout the month.

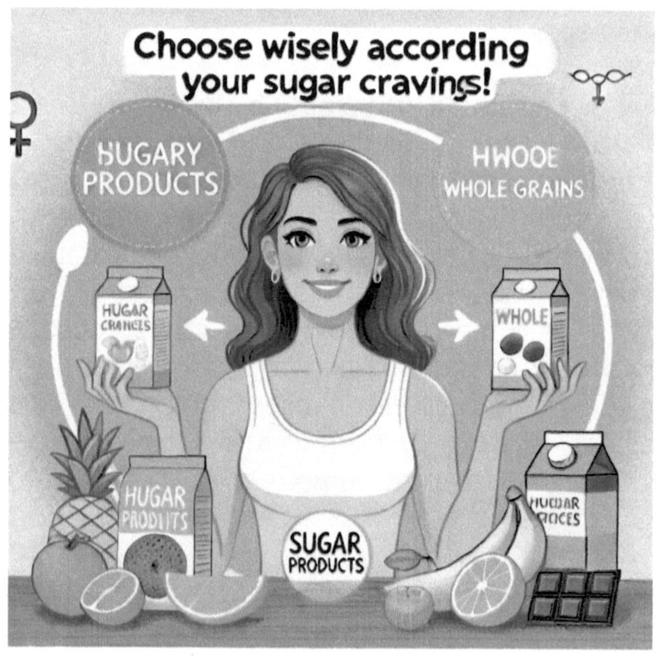

5

Mood Swings, Bloating, Cramps, Acne, Diarrhea, You Name It…

"The Symphony of Period Symptoms: An Unwanted Medley"

Unexplainable Cry, Mood Swings Before 3 Days**

Three days before her period, Maya finds herself crying over a commercial about puppies. It's not even a sad commercial; the puppies are playing happily in a field. But there she is, sobbing uncontrollably, and she knows exactly why—hormones.

Part 1: The Unexpected Tears

It's as if the universe has decided that every emotional trigger will hit at once. She cries because the weather is nice, because her coffee is too strong, because the cat looked at her funny. It's all too much, and yet, it's nothing at all. She knows she's being ridiculous, but she can't stop the tears.

Part 2: The Rollercoaster of Emotions

One moment, Maya is laughing hysterically at a meme her friend sent her. The next, she's angry because her favorite show ended on a cliffhanger. And then, out of nowhere, she's sad because she finished the last of her chocolate. It's like being on a rollercoaster with no off switch, and she's just along for the ride.

Part 3: Trying to Explain It

Maya tries to explain her mood swings to her Husband, who looks at her like she's speaking a foreign language. "It's just hormones," she says, as if that's supposed to make everything clear. But he doesn't get it, and honestly, she doesn't expect him to. It's not something you can understand unless you've lived it.

Part 4: The Humor in the Madness

Despite the emotional chaos, Maya can't help but find humor in the situation. She starts documenting her mood swings, turning them into funny anecdotes to share with her friends. They laugh with her because they've been there too, and sometimes, laughter is the best way to cope with the insanity.

Part 5: Embracing the Emotions

In the end, Maya realizes that these mood swings are just part of who she is. She can't control them, but she can choose how to react to them. So, she embraces the emotions, knowing that in a few days, they'll pass, and she'll be back to her normal, rational self—until next month, that is.

Let's face it—when it comes to period symptoms, Mother Nature didn't hold back. She gave us the full buffet of discomfort, and it's all-you-can-eat whether you're hungry for it or not. If periods were a concert, the symptoms would be the orchestra, playing in perfect (and painful) harmony. From mood swings to cramps, bloating to acne, and even the occasional surprise guest like diarrhea, it's a veritable symphony of suffering. So grab your popcorn—or, more accurately, your heating pad—and let's break down the greatest hits of period symptoms.

The Backup Singers: Cramps

Next in the lineup are cramps, the backup singers who are always a little too loud. You know they're coming—like that one annoying song on the radio that you can't escape—but that doesn't make them any easier to deal with. It starts with a dull ache, a warning sign that your uterus is about to go full-on rock concert mode. Then, just when you think you can handle it, the cramps hit you with the force of a thousand angry drummers.

These aren't just any cramps; these are the kind that make you question your life choices. You find yourself curled up in the fetal position, clutching your stomach as if you can somehow squeeze the pain away. Hot water bottles become your best friends, and you start wondering if you can legally marry ibuprofen. And let's not forget the creative ways you contort yourself to find some semblance of comfort—positions that would make a yoga instructor proud, or at least deeply confused.

On a daily basis approximate 17% female are on periods and crores of females are on their period and its not just the blood loss, hormones are also at pick and also during this period female has to prepare for exam, go to work and finish daily chores so there are definitely female around us are on period. So when you see a female is having mood swing you can guess she is on her periods.

Introducing Dolly: The Mood Swing Maestro

Meet Dolly, a woman who has mastered the art of navigating the emotional rollercoaster that comes with her period. She's the kind of person who can go from dancing around her living room to sobbing into her pillow, all within the span of an hour. But despite the wild swings, Dolly has learned to embrace the chaos with a sense of humor—and a whole lot of chocolate.

It's a Friday evening, and Dolly is feeling particularly energetic. She just got home from work, and her favorite song comes on the radio. Without a second thought, she cranks up the volume and starts dancing around her apartment like she's auditioning for a music video. She's happy, carefree, and completely in the moment. Nothing can bring her down.

But then, as quickly as the joy arrived, it fades. The song ends, and so does her mood. Dolly suddenly feels a wave of sadness wash over her, the kind that makes her want to crawl under a blanket and disappear. She sinks onto the couch, feeling the tears welling up. "What is wrong with me?" she wonders, even though she knows the answer. It's just the hormones, playing their usual tricks.

The Sadness That Won't Quit

Dolly grabs a tub of ice cream from the freezer—her go-to comfort food when the sadness hits. She curls up on the couch, spoon in hand, and starts to eat, hoping the sweetness will lift her spirits. But instead of feeling better, she finds herself getting even more emotional. The ice cream reminds her of the time she and her ex-Husband used to share late-night treats, and suddenly, she's spiraling into a full-on pity party.

"I miss him," she thinks, even though she knows she doesn't really. But that's the thing about period-induced sadness—it doesn't always make sense. It's like her brain is pulling up every sad memory she's ever had, just to make things worse.

And then, as if on cue, her best friend, VIsh, calls. VIsh knows all about Dolly's mood swings, and she's always ready to provide a much-needed distraction. "Hey, want to go out dancing tonight?" VIsh asks, her voice full of excitement.

Dolly hesitates, her mood still somewhere between melancholy and "leave me alone." But she knows that staying home will only make things worse. "Sure, why not?" she finally replies, forcing herself to sound more enthusiastic than she feels.

The Romance and Irritation Tango

The next day, Dolly is feeling a little better. She's rested, and the sadness from the night before has mostly lifted. She decides to spend the evening with her Husband, Ajay, hoping for a cozy night in. They order takeout, watch a movie, and everything seems perfect. Dolly feels a surge of affection for Ajay, and they start to cuddle on the couch, the mood turning romantic.

But as things heat up, something shifts. Suddenly, Dolly feels irritated. The way Ajay's hand brushes against her skin, the sound of his breathing—everything is getting on her nerves. She tries to push the feelings aside, not wanting to ruin the moment, but it's no use. The irritation is too strong.

"Is everything okay?" Ajay asks, noticing her sudden change in demeanor.

Dolly sighs, frustrated with herself. "Yeah, I'm just... I don't know, it's the hormones," she admits, pulling away slightly.

Ajay, ever patient, nods in understanding. "Do you want to stop?" he asks gently.

Dolly nods, feeling both relieved and guilty. "Yeah, I think I just need a minute."

They sit in silence for a moment, the romantic mood all but evaporated. Dolly can't help but feel frustrated—why does her body have to sabotage her like this? But then Ajay does something that makes her laugh. He starts to mimic the exaggerated dance moves she was doing earlier, waving his arms around like a cartoon character. It's so ridiculous that Dolly can't help but burst into laughter, the tension melting away.

"See, I knew I could make you smile," Ajay says with a grin.

Dolly shakes her head, still laughing. "You're ridiculous, but thank you," she says, feeling a little better.

The Relatable Rollercoaster

Dolly's experiences with mood swings are something every woman can relate to. Whether it's going from happy to sad in a matter of minutes, feeling the sudden need to sleep for hours, or being overwhelmed by irritation just when things are getting romantic, these emotional ups and downs are all too familiar.

But what makes Dolly's story so relatable is that she doesn't let these mood swings define her. She might feel like she's on an emotional rollercoaster, but she's learned to ride the waves with humor and a bit of grace. And most importantly, she knows she's not alone—every woman has been there at one time or another.

So, the next time you find yourself dancing one minute and crying the next, or loving someone deeply only to feel irritated by them moments later, just remember Dolly. Remember that it's okay to feel all the feelings, to let your emotions dance around you like a wild, unpredictable partner. Because in the end, it's all part of the beautiful, messy experience of being human—and being a woman.

And if all else fails, there's always chocolate, a good friend, and maybe a little ridiculous dancing to help you through.

The Roadies: Bloating

And then there's bloating—the roadies of the period symptoms concert. They show up uninvited, set up camp, and make themselves at home. Suddenly, your pants don't fit, your stomach feels like a water balloon, and you're pretty sure you've gained five pounds overnight. But it's not just the physical discomfort; it's the psychological warfare that bloating wages on your self-esteem.

You look in the mirror and wonder who that puffy stranger is staring back at you. Your once flat(ish) stomach has been replaced by a ballooning monstrosity, and you feel like you're wearing a permanent flotation device. But the worst part? Knowing that it's all just temporary. You're not really gaining weight, but your body is convinced otherwise, and it's making sure you know it.

The Drummer: Acne

Acne is the drummer of the group, pounding away with relentless energy. Just when you think you've got your skin under control, your hormones decide to throw a wrench in the works. You wake up one morning, look in the mirror, and boom—there it is. That big, angry pimple right in the middle of your forehead, like a flashing neon sign that says, "Hey, I'm on my period!"

But it's not just one pimple, oh no. Acne during your period likes to come in clusters, as if your skin is having a breakout party and forgot to invite you. It's like being a teenager all over again, only now you have the added bonus of wrinkles to contend with. You try every remedy under the sun—creams, masks, even toothpaste in a pinch—but nothing seems to work. All you can do is wait it out and hope that your skin decides to cooperate again once the hormonal storm passes.

The Bass Player: Diarrhea

Finally, we have diarrhea—the bass player of period symptoms, rumbling away in the background, sometimes subtly, sometimes not. For reasons that still baffle scientists, your period has a way of messing with your digestive system. One day, you're constipated; the next, you're running to the bathroom every five minutes. It's like your body can't decide whether to hold onto everything or let it all go, and it's taking you along for the ride.

Diarrhea is one of those symptoms that no one likes to talk about, but let's be real—it's a thing, and it's not fun. You find yourself planning your day around bathroom access, praying that you don't have a surprise attack while you're out in public. And when it does hit, it's with the subtlety of a freight train. You start questioning everything you've eaten in the past 24 hours, wondering if it's the culprit, when deep down you know it's just your period being its usual, unpredictable self.

The Encore: The Unexpected Combo

Just when you think the concert is over, your period decides to hit you with an encore—an unexpected combo of all the symptoms at once. You're bloated, cramping, emotional, and breaking out, all while dealing with digestive issues that would make a gastroenterologist shudder. It's the perfect storm of discomfort, and there's no way to escape it.

But here's the thing: you've survived it before, and you'll survive it again. Because despite all the misery that period symptoms bring, there's a weird sense of camaraderie in knowing that every woman out there is dealing with the same thing. We're all in this together, experiencing the same symphony of symptoms month after month.

And as much as we may hate it, there's something

empowering about being able to handle it all. We may complain (and rightfully so), but we still get up, go to work, take care of our responsibilities, and live our lives, all while battling an internal orchestra of discomfort. We're warriors, even when we don't feel like it.

So next time you're in the throes of period symptoms, remember—you're not alone, and you're stronger than you think. And if all else fails, a little humor and a lot of chocolate can go a long way.

6

Vacation, Birthday, Marriage, Temple, and U Get Ur Period

"Periods: The Ultimate Event Crasher"

If there's one thing that periods are great at, it's their impeccable sense of timing. Not in a good way, of course. No, periods have a unique ability to show up at the most inconvenient, untimely, and downright annoying moments possible. It's like they have a built-in radar for when you've planned something special, and they decide to crash the party just for fun. Vacation? Period. Birthday? Period. Wedding? Period. Visiting a temple? Yep, you guessed it—period.

The Vacation Saboteur

Picture this: You've been planning your dream vacation for months. You've booked the perfect hotel, packed your cutest outfits, and created an itinerary that includes plenty of relaxation, adventure, and fun. Everything is ready, and you're counting down the days with excitement. And then, like clockwork, your period arrives the day before you're set to leave. Cue the collective groan of frustration.

Instead of lounging on the beach in that new bikini, you're suddenly more concerned about whether your tampon will hold up through a swim in the ocean. You were looking forward to sipping cocktails by the pool, but now you're dealing with cramps that make you want to curl up in a ball instead. And let's not even talk about the bloating—because nothing says "vacation ready" like feeling like you've swallowed a beach ball.

Your carefully planned outfits? Replaced with the most comfortable, flowy clothes you can find, because let's be real—there's no way you're squeezing into those cute shorts when your stomach is throwing a bloated tantrum. And that hiking adventure you were so excited about? Postponed, because the idea of tackling a mountain while your uterus is waging war sounds like the worst idea ever.

But the worst part? The constant worry about leaks. You're on high alert, checking and double-checking that everything is in place, praying that you don't have a wardrobe malfunction in the middle of your vacation photoshoot. And just when you start to relax and think you've got it under control, another wave of cramps hits, reminding you that your period isn't done messing with your plans.

The Birthday Ruiner

Birthdays are supposed to be all about you—your day to celebrate, indulge, and be spoiled rotten. But if your period has anything to say about it, it's going to make sure that your special day comes with a side of discomfort. Forget about enjoying that fancy birthday dinner; you're too busy battling bloating and trying to ignore the fact that your dress feels about two sizes too small.

You were hoping to spend the day surrounded by friends, laughing and having fun, but instead, you're secretly wishing you could just go home, put on your comfiest pajamas, and binge-watch your favorite shows with a heating pad on your stomach. The cake you were so excited to eat? Now it's just another thing that might upset your already sensitive stomach. And don't even get me started on the surprise party your friends planned—because nothing says "happy birthday" like having to excuse yourself every hour to deal with your period.

Of course, your friends and family mean well. They want you to have the best day possible, and you don't want to spoil the fun. So, you put on a brave face, smile through the discomfort, and try to enjoy the day as much as you can. But deep down, you can't help but feel a little cheated. Why, of all days, did your period have to show up now?

The Wedding Crasher

Ah, weddings—the ultimate celebration of love, commitment, and, if you're lucky, a killer open bar. Whether it's your wedding or someone else's, weddings are supposed to be joyful occasions filled with laughter, dancing, and memories that will last a lifetime. But if your period has anything to say about it, those memories will also include a healthy dose of cramps, mood swings, and a whole lot of bathroom breaks.

If it's your own wedding, the stakes are even higher. You've spent months—maybe even years—planning every detail, from the flowers to the seating chart. You've found the perfect dress, the perfect venue, and the perfect playlist. Everything is set for the most magical day of your life. And then, like a cruel joke, your period decides to make an appearance.

Suddenly, the dress that fit you like a glove in the final fitting is now a bit too snug, thanks to bloating. You're trying to enjoy the ceremony, but all you can think about is whether you'll make it through without needing a bathroom break. And those gorgeous heels you splurged on? They're no match for the cramps that make you want to kick them off and dance barefoot instead.

If you're a guest at someone else's wedding, the challenges are different but no less frustrating. You're trying to be present, to enjoy the celebration, but your period has other plans. The reception becomes a balancing act between enjoying yourself and making sure you don't have a wardrobe malfunction on the dance floor. And the worst part? Trying to discreetly carry your period supplies in a tiny clutch that barely fits your phone, let alone anything else.

The Temple Visit That Almost Wasn't

There's something sacred and serene about visiting a temple—a place to reflect, to find peace, and to connect with something greater than yourself. But if your period has anything to say about it, that peace is going to come with a side of stress. For many, visiting a temple while on your period is a no-go due to cultural or religious beliefs. So, what do you do when you've planned a visit, and your period decides to show up uninvited?

You might find yourself frantically calculating dates, trying to figure out if you can reschedule the visit or if you'll have to sit this one out. If you do decide to go, you're navigating a minefield of emotions—guilt, anxiety, and frustration—while trying to maintain a sense of reverence and respect. It's a delicate balance, and it's one that your period seems determined to upset.

And even if you're not restricted from entering the temple, the physical discomfort of your period can make the visit far less peaceful

7
Food You Should Eat During Periods

"The Period Diet: Cravings, Comfort Food, and a Touch of Nutrition"

Let's talk about food. Specifically, the food you should eat during your period. Now, if we're being completely honest, there's a big difference between what we *should* eat and what we *want* to eat when Aunt Flo comes to visit. Because let's face it—when your uterus is throwing a temper tantrum, your brain is screaming for chocolate, chips, and anything that's deep-fried and smothered in cheese.

But somewhere in the middle of those cravings and nutritional advice, there's a sweet spot. A place where you can find comfort in your food while also giving your body what it needs to survive the monthly rollercoaster. So, let's dive into the funny, the relatable, and the downright necessary foods that should be on your period menu.

The Craving Conundrum: Chocolate and Chips

Picture this: It's the first day of your period, and you're curled up on the couch in your comfiest pajamas, clutching a heating pad like it's a lifeline. Your cramps are in full swing, and your mood is somewhere between "don't talk to me" and "I might cry if you look at me the wrong way." Naturally, your thoughts turn to food—specifically, chocolate. Because if there's one thing that can make this day better, it's a big, gooey brownie or a handful of your favorite chocolate candy.

So, you raid the kitchen, searching for that sweet, sweet relief. And there it is, tucked away in the back of the pantry—a bar of dark chocolate, practically calling your name. You break off a piece, savoring the rich, bittersweet flavor as it melts in your mouth. For a moment, the cramps don't seem so bad, and your mood lifts just a little. It's like a hug for your soul.

But then, the craving hits again, this time for something salty. Chips! Yes, the perfect complement to your chocolate. You grab a bag and start munching away, alternating between bites of chocolate and handfuls of chips. It's not the most balanced meal, but hey, it's your period—you deserve to indulge a little.

The Comfort Food Quandary: Mac and Cheese vs. Nutrient-Packed Meals

Let's be real—comfort food is a period essential. There's something about a warm, cheesy bowl of mac and cheese that just makes everything feel a little bit better. It's like a security blanket for your insides, wrapping you up in creamy, carb-loaded goodness. But while mac and cheese might be your go-to comfort food, it's not exactly the best choice for keeping your period symptoms in check.

Enter the Period Power Bowl—a meal that's as comforting as it is nutritious. Picture this: a bowl filled with quinoa (hello, whole grains), topped with sautéed spinach (for that much-needed iron), roasted sweet potatoes (a natural source of magnesium), and a drizzle of olive oil (healthy fats to help balance your hormones). Add a sprinkle of feta cheese and a handful of walnuts, and you've got yourself a meal that's both delicious and good for your period woes.

Now, I know what you're thinking: "That sounds great, but it's not mac and cheese." And you're right—nothing can truly replace the cheesy, gooey goodness of your favorite comfort food

Top of Form
Bottom of Form

The Touching Tale: Grandma's Period Soup

Speaking of giving your body love, let me tell you a story about my grandmother. She was a woman who believed that food was medicine, and she had a recipe for just about every ailment. For headaches, she made ginger tea. For colds, it was chicken soup with extra garlic. And for periods, she had her special period soup—a concoction of ingredients that she swore would make everything better.

The soup was simple—just a few basic ingredients: chicken broth, a handful of greens, a squeeze of lemon, and a secret blend of spices that she never revealed. But somehow, it worked. Whenever I had my period and the cramps were unbearable, she'd make me a bowl of that soup. The warmth would soothe my aching belly, the greens would give me a boost of energy, and the lemon would lift my spirits. But more than that, it was the love she put into making it that made me feel better.

I remember one particularly bad period when I was in my early teens. I was doubled over in pain, feeling like the world was ending, when Grandma walked in with a steaming bowl of her period soup. She sat down next to me, placed the bowl in my hands, and said, "Eat this, sweetheart. It'll help, I promise." I took a sip, and though it didn't cure my cramps, it did make me feel just a little bit stronger. It was like Grandma had poured all her love and care into that bowl, and with every bite, I felt less alone in my pain.

Years later, I found myself making that same soup for a friend who was struggling with her own period symptoms. I didn't have Grandma's secret spice blend, but I did my best to recreate the recipe from memory. As I watched my friend take her first sip, I saw a familiar look of relief wash over her face. It wasn't just the soup—it was the act of caring, of nurturing, that made the difference.

The Balance: Indulging and Nourishing

So, what's the moral of this story? It's simple: during your period, it's okay to indulge in your cravings, but don't forget to nourish your body too. There's room for both chocolate and spinach, for mac and cheese and quinoa. It's all about balance—finding that sweet spot where you can satisfy your cravings while also giving your body the nutrients it needs to handle your period like a champ.

So next time you're stocking up for that time of the month, grab a bar of your favorite chocolate, but maybe also pick up some leafy greens, a sweet potato, and a bag of walnuts. You don't have to choose between comfort and nutrition—you can have both. And who knows? You might just find that the foods you should eat during your period are also the ones you actually want to eat.

And if all else fails, there's always Grandma's period soup. It might not be a miracle cure, but it's made with love—and sometimes, that's exactly what you need.

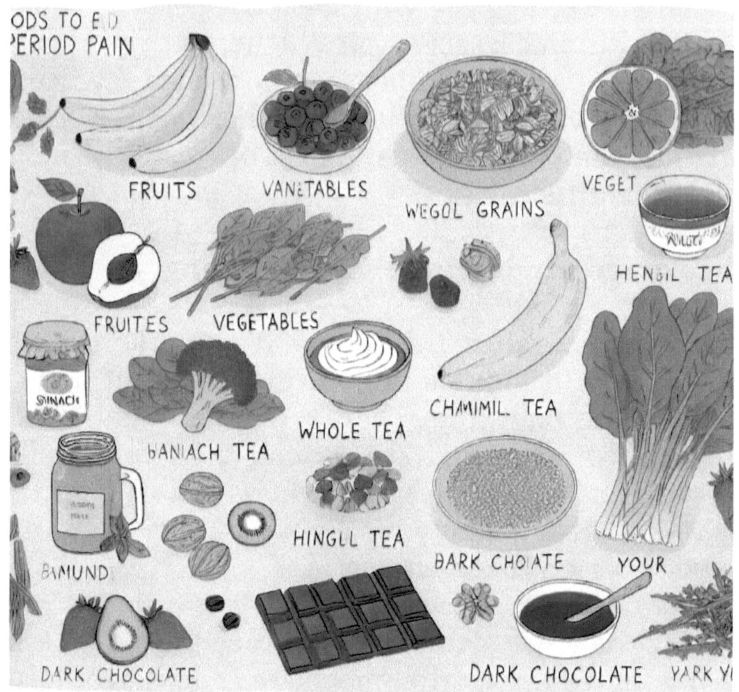

Food You Should Eat During Periods

"The Period Diet: Cravings, Comfort Food, and a Touch of Nutrition"

Let's talk about food. Specifically, the food you should eat during your period. Now, if we're being completely honest, there's a big difference between what we *should* eat and what we *want* to eat when Aunt Flo comes to visit. Because let's face it—when your uterus is throwing a temper tantrum, your brain is screaming for chocolate, chips, and anything that's deep-fried and smothered in cheese.

But somewhere in the middle of those cravings and nutritional advice, there's a sweet spot. A place where you can find comfort in your food while also giving your body what it needs to survive the monthly rollercoaster. So, let's dive into the funny, the relatable, and the downright necessary foods that should be on your period menu.

The Craving Conundrum: Chocolate and Chips

Picture this: It's the first day of your period, and you're curled up on the couch in your comfiest pajamas, clutching a heating pad like it's a lifeline. Your cramps are in full swing, and your mood is somewhere between "don't talk to me" and "I might cry if you look at me the wrong way." Naturally, your thoughts turn to food—specifically, chocolate. Because if there's one thing that can make this day better, it's a big, gooey brownie or a handful of your favorite chocolate candy.

So, you raid the kitchen, searching for that sweet, sweet relief. And there it is, tucked away in the back of the pantry—a bar of dark chocolate, practically calling your name. You break off a piece, savoring the rich, bittersweet flavor as it melts in your mouth. For a moment, the cramps don't seem so bad, and your mood lifts just a little. It's like a hug for your soul.

But then, the craving hits again, this time for something salty. Chips! Yes, the perfect complement to your chocolate. You grab a bag and start munching away, alternating between bites of chocolate and handfuls of chips. It's not the most balanced meal, but hey, it's your period—you deserve to indulge a little.

As you sit there, surrounded by wrappers and crumbs, you start to wonder if there's a better way. A way to satisfy your cravings while also giving your body the nutrients it needs to fight off those nasty period symptoms. And that's when you remember the article you read about period-friendly foods. You know, the one that mentioned things like leafy greens and whole grains—foods that are supposed to help with bloating, cramps, and mood swings.

You chuckle to yourself, imagining a version of you that actually reaches for a salad instead of chips. "Yeah, right," you think, but deep down, you know there's some truth to it. Because as much as you love chocolate and chips, you also know that your body might just feel a little better if you mixed in some actual nutrients.

The Comfort Food Quandary: Mac and Cheese vs. Nutrient-Packed Meals

Let's be real—comfort food is a period essential. There's something about a warm, cheesy bowl of mac and cheese that just makes everything feel a little bit better. It's like a security blanket for your insides, wrapping you up in creamy, carb-loaded goodness. But while mac and cheese might be your go-to comfort food, it's not exactly the best choice for keeping your period symptoms in check.

Enter the Period Power Bowl—a meal that's as comforting as it is nutritious. Picture this: a bowl filled with quinoa (hello, whole grains), topped with sautéed spinach (for that much-needed iron), roasted sweet potatoes (a natural source of magnesium), and a drizzle of olive oil (healthy fats to help balance your hormones). Add a sprinkle of feta cheese and a handful of walnuts, and you've got yourself a meal that's both delicious and good for your period woes.

Now, I know what you're thinking: "That sounds great, but it's not mac and cheese." And you're right—nothing can truly replace the cheesy, gooey goodness of your favorite comfort food

Top of Form
Bottom of Form

The Touching Tale: Grandma's Period Soup

Speaking of giving your body love, let me tell you a story

about my grandmother. She was a woman who believed that food was medicine, and she had a recipe for just about every ailment. For headaches, she made ginger tea. For colds, it was chicken soup with extra garlic. And for periods, she had her special period soup—a concoction of ingredients that she swore would make everything better.

The soup was simple—just a few basic ingredients: chicken broth, a handful of greens, a squeeze of lemon, and a secret blend of spices that she never revealed. But somehow, it worked. Whenever I had my period and the cramps were unbearable, she'd make me a bowl of that soup. The warmth would soothe my aching belly, the greens would give me a boost of energy, and the lemon would lift my spirits. But more than that, it was the love she put into making it that made me feel better.

I remember one particularly bad period when I was in my early teens. I was doubled over in pain, feeling like the world was ending, when Grandma walked in with a steaming bowl of her period soup. She sat down next to me, placed the bowl in my hands, and said, "Eat this, sweetheart. It'll help, I promise." I took a sip, and though it didn't cure my cramps, it did make me feel just a little bit stronger. It was like Grandma had poured all her love and care into that bowl, and with every bite, I felt less alone in my pain.

Years later, I found myself making that same soup for a friend who was struggling with her own period symptoms. I didn't have Grandma's secret spice blend, but I did my best to recreate the recipe from memory. As I watched my friend take her first sip, I saw a familiar look of relief wash over her face. It wasn't just the soup—it was the act of caring, of nurturing, that made the difference.

The Balance: Indulging and Nourishing

So, what's the moral of this story? It's simple: during your period, it's okay to indulge in your cravings, but don't forget to nourish your body too. There's room for both chocolate and spinach, for mac and cheese and quinoa. It's all about balance—finding that sweet spot where you can satisfy your cravings while also giving your body the nutrients it needs to handle your period like a champ.

So next time you're stocking up for that time of the month, grab a bar of your favorite chocolate, but maybe also pick up some leafy greens, a sweet potato, and a bag of walnuts. You don't have to choose between comfort and nutrition—you can have both. And who knows? You might just find that the foods you should eat during your period are also the ones you actually want to eat.

And if all else fails, there's always Grandma's period soup. It might not be a miracle cure, but it's made with love—and sometimes, that's exactly what you need.

8

Periods and Exercise

"The Love-Hate Relationship Between Periods and Exercise"

Exercise and periods—two things that, on the surface, seem like they should never mix. After all, who in their right mind would choose to engage in physical activity when their uterus feels like it's auditioning for a role in a horror movie? But here's the thing: despite the discomfort, the bloating, and the general feeling of "I'd rather be in bed," exercise can actually be one of the best things you do for yourself during your period.

Of course, getting to that point—where you actually *want* to exercise—is a journey in itself, filled with plenty of humorous (and sometimes painful) moments. So let's dive into the love-hate relationship between periods and exercise, and why, despite everything, it's worth lacing up those sneakers.

The Reluctant Athlete: Dragging Yourself to the Gym

Let's start with the obvious: the days leading up to your period are usually not the time when you're feeling your most athletic. Instead, you're more likely to be found curled up on the couch, binge-watching Netflix with a bag of chips in hand. The thought of going to the gym, or even just taking a walk, feels like a Herculean task. Your body is tired, your mood is in the gutter, and the last thing you want to do is break a sweat.

But here's where the irony kicks in: those days when you feel the least like exercising are often the days when you need it the most. Exercise, as it turns out, is like the ultimate period paradox. You don't want to do it, but when you do, you feel so much better.

So, how do you motivate yourself to actually get moving? Sometimes it's sheer willpower, sometimes it's the promise of treating yourself afterward, and sometimes it's just the knowledge that exercise can help ease those dreaded period symptoms. But more often than not, it's a combination of all three—along with a fair amount of internal pep-talking as you drag yourself to the gym.

The First Few Minutes: Why Did I Think This Was a Good Idea?

You've made it to the gym. Great! But as soon as you start warming up, the doubts creep in. "Why did I think this was a good idea?" you wonder as you step onto the treadmill. Your body feels heavy, your legs are sluggish, and every step seems to echo the voice in your head telling you to quit and go home.

But let me tell u my experience

My Mrs. India Fitness Journey

Participating in the Mrs. India Competition in December 2023 was an exhilarating experience that tested my physical endurance and mental strength. During the workout day, all participants were called early in the morning for a rigorous exercise session. Despite taking my medication beforehand, I felt an inexplicable surge of energy and determination coursing through my body—a sense of divine strength that seemed to guide me through each movement. Though some exercises were challenging, I gave my best effort and surprised myself by completing them. My squats may not have been perfect, but I did them with resilience. I managed to hold a

30-second plank, performed high knees, and even attempted burpees. This experience reminded me that with the right mindset and perseverance, we can push our limits and achieve what we once thought impossible.

The first few minutes of exercising on your period are often the hardest. You're battling not just physical discomfort, but also the mental resistance that comes with knowing you could be at home, doing absolutely nothing. But here's the trick: if you can push through those first few minutes, something amazing happens. Your body starts to warm up, your muscles loosen, and suddenly, it doesn't feel so bad.

In fact, by the time you've finished your warm-up, you might even find that you're starting to enjoy yourself. Your mood lifts, the endorphins kick in, and for the first time all day, you feel like maybe—just maybe—you're glad you decided to work out. It's like a little victory over your period, a reminder that you're stronger than you think.

The Exercise Choices: To Yoga or Not to Yoga?

When it comes to exercising during your period, not all workouts are created equal. Some activities—like gentle yoga or a brisk walk—can feel like a soothing balm for your aching body. Others—like an intense spin class or heavy lifting—might make you want to curl up in a ball and cry. The key is to listen to your body and choose an exercise that feels right for you.

Yoga is often touted as the ultimate period workout, and for good reason. The gentle stretching, deep breathing, and focus on relaxation can do wonders for your cramps, your mood, and your overall sense of well-being. Plus, there's something about rolling out your mat, lighting a candle, and just focusing on yourself for a while that feels incredibly nourishing.

But if yoga isn't your thing, don't worry—there are plenty of other options. A light jog, a swim, or even just a walk in the park can all help to ease period symptoms and boost your mood. The key is to keep it low-impact and not to push yourself too hard. Remember, you're not trying to break any records—you're just trying to feel a little bit better.

And then there are those days when your body says, "Nope, not today." On those days, it's perfectly okay to skip the workout, stay in bed, and take care of yourself in other ways. Exercise can be incredibly beneficial during your period, but it's not a requirement. If your body needs rest, give it rest. The gym will still be there tomorrow.

The Post-Workout Glow: I Did It!

You've made it through your workout. You're sweaty, tired, and maybe even a little sore, but you did it. And as you head home, you realize something: you feel good. Your cramps have eased up, your mood has improved, and your body feels lighter. It's that post-workout glow—the one that's even more satisfying because you know you had every reason to skip the gym, and yet you didn't.

There's a sense of pride that comes with exercising during your period. It's not easy, and it's certainly not always fun, but it's a reminder that you're capable of more than you think. Your period might slow you down, but it doesn't stop you. And that's something to celebrate.

The moral of the story? Know your limits. Sometimes, a gentle walk or a bit of yoga is all you need. And sometimes, it's okay to skip the gym entirely. Exercise can be a great way to manage period symptoms, but it's not a one-size-fits-all solution. Listen to your body, and do what feels right for you.

The Conclusion: Finding What Works for You

In the end, the relationship between periods and exercise is a personal one. For some, exercise is a lifeline during their period—a way to feel better, both physically and mentally. For others, it's a struggle to even consider lacing up their shoes. And that's okay.

What matters is finding what works for you. Maybe it's a gentle yoga session, a walk in the park, or even just stretching at home. Maybe it's a full workout at the gym, or maybe it's taking the week off to rest. There's no right or wrong way to handle exercise during your period—only what feels good for you.

So next time your period rolls around, don't be afraid to experiment. Try different workouts, see how your body responds, and give yourself permission to rest if that's what you need. Because at the end of the day, exercise during your period is about taking care of yourself—whatever that looks like for you.

And remember: you're strong, you're capable, and you've got this—period or not.

Effects of Exercises .... Notes from Experts

1. **Releases Endorphins**

When you exercise, your body releases endorphins, which are natural painkillers and mood boosters. Endorphins can help counteract the pain signals from cramps, making you feel better both physically and emotionally.

2. **Improves Blood Circulation**

Exercise increases blood flow, which can help reduce the severity of cramps by delivering more oxygen to your muscles, including those in your uterus. Better circulation can also help reduce bloating and fatigue. (I experienced it personally)

3. **Reduces Stress**

Physical activity is a great way to manage stress, which can sometimes exacerbate period symptoms. Reducing stress can lead to fewer mood swings and less overall discomfort during your period. (I also explored dancing at home during my periods when pain stopped immediately after medicines)

4. **Balances Hormones**

Regular exercise can help regulate your hormones, which may reduce the intensity of period symptoms over time. It's not a quick fix, but consistent physical activity can contribute to a more balanced menstrual cycle.

5. **Eases Bloating**

Movement, especially gentle exercise like walking or yoga, can help alleviate bloating by promoting digestion and reducing water retention.

6. **Supports Better Sleep**

Exercise can improve your sleep quality, which is often disrupted during your period. Better sleep can help you feel more rested and better able to cope with period pain.

What Type of Exercise Is Best?

- **Low-Impact Exercises:** Activities like walking, swimming, or cycling are gentle on the body and can be effective in relieving period pain without overexerting yourself.

- **Yoga:** Certain yoga poses, especially those that focus on stretching and relaxation, can be particularly helpful for easing cramps and reducing stress.

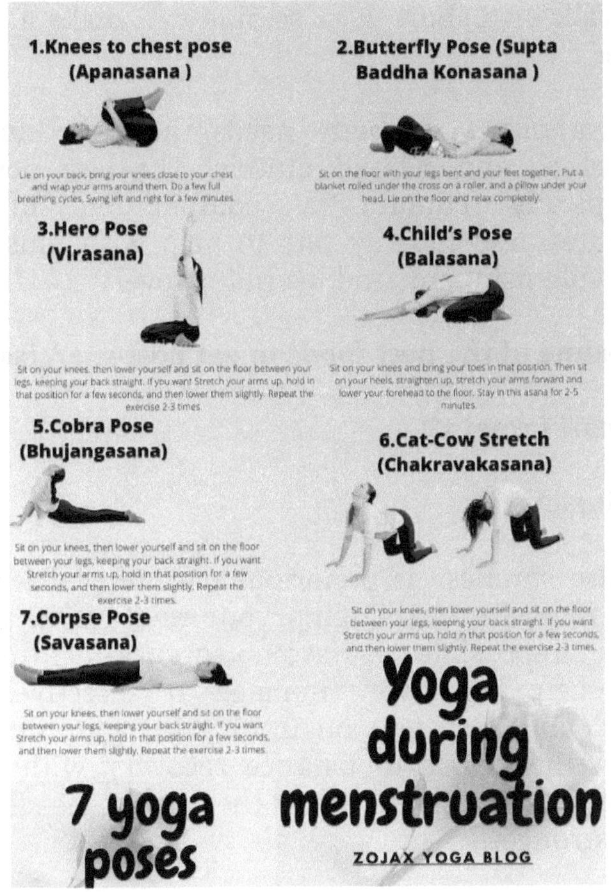

When to Avoid Exercise

While exercise can be beneficial, it's important to listen to your body. If your period symptoms are particularly severe or you're feeling extremely fatigued, it might be best to opt for rest instead of a workout. Also, avoid high-intensity workouts if they exacerbate your symptoms or if you're feeling lightheaded or dizzy.

In summary, while exercise might not be the first thing you want to do during your period, it can actually be an effective way to ease pain and improve your overall well-being. Even a gentle walk or a short yoga session can make a significant difference.

After a workout, your body needs the right nutrients to recover, refuel, and rebuild muscle. The best post-exercise foods typically contain a combination of protein, carbohydrates, and healthy fats to help with muscle repair, glycogen replenishment, and overall recovery.

Here are some of the best foods to eat post-exercise:

1. **Lean Protein**

Conclusion

Post-exercise soreness is a normal part of physical activity, especially if you're challenging your muscles in new ways. While it's impossible to avoid soreness entirely, these strategies can help you manage it effectively, reduce discomfort, and keep you on track with your fitness goals. Remember, the key is to balance recovery with continued movement—allowing your body the time it needs to repair and grow stronger.

9

Adult Diapers and Tampons: Myths, Facts, and the Science Behind Usage

The Quiet Revolution: Embracing Adult Diapers and Tampons

When it comes to managing periods, there's no one-size-fits-all solution. Every woman has her own preferences, needs, and comfort levels, which is why it's so important to have a variety of options. Two of the most discussed—and sometimes misunderstood—options are adult diapers and tampons. Both have their own set of benefits, myths, and scientific backing, but they also carry a fair share of stigma. In this chapter, we'll explore the truth behind these products, debunk some common myths, and take a closer look at the science behind their use.

Adult Diapers: A Lifesaver for Heavy Flow Days

For many women, the idea of using an adult diaper during their period might seem extreme or even embarrassing. But the truth is, adult diapers can be a game-changer, especially for those with heavy menstrual flow, overnight protection needs, or specific medical conditions.

Benefits:

- **Leak Protection:** Adult diapers provide full coverage, reducing the risk of leaks, particularly during the night or on heavy flow days. This can be especially comforting if you're tired of waking up to stained sheets or worrying about accidents while you're out and about.

- **Comfort:** Modern adult diapers are designed with comfort in mind. They're made from soft, breathable materials that wick away moisture, keeping you dry and comfortable for hours.

- **Convenience:** For those with busy schedules or limited access to bathrooms, adult diapers can offer peace of mind, knowing you won't need to change as frequently as with pads or tampons.

Myths Debunked:

- **"Adult Diapers Are Only for Incontinence":** While they are commonly associated with incontinence, adult diapers are a perfectly valid option for period protection, especially for women who experience very heavy periods or need extra coverage during sleep.

- **"They're Uncomfortable and Bulky":** This might have been true decades ago, but modern adult diapers are designed to be discreet and comfortable, with a slim fit that's barely noticeable under clothing.

Scientific View:

The technology behind adult diapers has come a long way. The absorbent materials used in these products, such as superabsorbent polymers, are highly effective at locking in moisture and preventing leaks. The design also ensures that moisture is drawn away from the skin, reducing the risk of irritation and infections. For women with medical conditions like endometriosis or those going through postpartum recovery, adult diapers can provide an extra layer of protection and comfort.

Tampons: A Trusted Companion for Active Days

Tampons have been a staple in menstrual care for decades, offering women a discreet, convenient way to manage their periods. Despite their popularity, tampons are often surrounded by myths and misconceptions that can make some women hesitant to use them.

Benefits:

- **Freedom of Movement:** Tampons allow you to move freely and participate in activities like swimming, running, or yoga without worrying about leaks or discomfort. They're ideal for women with active lifestyles.

- **Discreetness:** Tampons are small and easy to carry, making them a discreet option for period protection. They're also virtually invisible when worn, allowing you to wear any outfit without fear of visible lines or bulk.

- **Less Odor:** Because tampons are worn internally, they help minimize the odor that can sometimes accompany menstrual flow, giving you added confidence.

Myths Debunked:

- **"Tampons Are Unsafe and Cause Toxic Shock Syndrome (TSS)":** While TSS is a serious condition, it's extremely rare, and the risk can be minimized by using tampons correctly. This includes choosing the lowest absorbency needed, changing tampons regularly (every 4-8 hours), and following the manufacturer's instructions.

- **"Tampons Can Get Lost Inside Your Body":** This is a common fear, but it's impossible for a tampon to get lost inside you. The tampon is held in place by your vaginal muscles, and the string remains outside for easy removal.

Scientific View:

Tampons are made from either cotton, rayon, or a blend of both. They work by absorbing menstrual fluid before it leaves the body, which can be more comfortable for some women than external products like pads. The risk of TSS, while often highlighted, is actually very low, especially with proper use. The key is to use the right absorbency for your flow and to change tampons regularly to prevent bacterial growth.

Research also shows that tampons, when used correctly, are safe and effective. They don't interfere with the body's natural processes, and for many women, they offer a level of convenience and comfort that's unmatched by other menstrual products.

Myths and Misconceptions: Separating Fact from Fiction

Beyond the specific myths surrounding adult diapers and tampons, there are some general misconceptions about menstrual products that need to be addressed.

Myth 1: "Using Tampons Can Affect Your Virginity"

This is a common concern in some cultures, but it's important to clarify that using a tampon does not affect virginity. Virginity is a social and cultural concept, not a physical condition. While inserting a tampon might stretch or tear the hymen, this doesn't equate to losing virginity.

Myth 2: "Adult Diapers Are for the Elderly"

As discussed earlier, adult diapers are versatile and can be used by anyone who needs extra protection, regardless of age. They're particularly useful for women with heavy periods, postpartum recovery, or other medical conditions that cause heavy bleeding.

Myth 3: "Tampons and Adult Diapers Are Bad for the Environment"

While it's true that disposable menstrual products contribute to waste, there are more eco-friendly options available. Many brands now offer organic, biodegradable tampons, and there are reusable options like cloth pads or menstrual cups that can significantly reduce your environmental footprint.

The Science of Comfort and Protection

Both tampons and adult diapers have been rigorously tested to ensure they're safe, comfortable, and effective. Modern designs focus on using materials that are both absorbent and breathable, reducing the risk of irritation and infection.

Tampons, for instance, are designed to absorb fluid while minimizing contact with the vaginal walls, which helps maintain the natural pH balance. Meanwhile, adult diapers are engineered to wick moisture away from the skin, keeping you dry and comfortable even during heavy flow days.

From a scientific standpoint, both products offer unique advantages that can make managing your period easier and more comfortable. The key is to find what works best for your body and your lifestyle

Conclusion: Choosing What's Right for You

At the end of the day, whether you choose tampons, adult diapers, or another menstrual product entirely, what matters most is your comfort and confidence. Every woman's body is different, and what works for one person might not work for another. It's important to try different options and see what suits you best.

Don't let myths or misconceptions stop you from exploring new products. Both tampons and adult diapers offer valuable benefits that can make your period a little more manageable, so embrace the choices available to you and pick what makes you feel empowered.

And remember, there's no right or wrong way to manage your period—only what works for you.

This chapter provides a balanced overview of adult diapers and tampons, addressing common myths, highlighting their benefits, and incorporating scientific insights. It aims to empower readers to make informed choices about their menstrual care.

Here are some of the key benefits of using menstrual cups:

1. **Cost-Effective**

- **Long-Term Savings:** Although menstrual cups have a higher upfront cost (usually between Rs249/- and Rs625/-) they can last for several years with proper care. This makes them far more cost-effective over time compared to disposable pads and tampons, which need to be purchased every month.

2. **Environmentally Friendly**

- **Reduces Waste:** Menstrual cups are reusable, which significantly reduces the amount of waste generated from disposable period products. A single cup can be used for up to 10 years, preventing thousands of tampons or pads from ending up in landfills.

- **Less Packaging:** Since you only need one cup, you also reduce the packaging waste associated with disposable products.

3. **Longer Wear Time**

- **Up to 12 Hours of Protection:** Menstrual cups can be worn for up to 12 hours, depending on your flow, which is longer than most tampons or pads. This means fewer changes throughout the day and more convenience, especially when you're out and about or during overnight use.

4. **Health Benefits**

- **No Exposure to Chemicals:** Menstrual cups are typically made from medical-grade silicone, latex, or rubber and do not contain the bleach, dyes, and chemicals that are sometimes found in tampons and pads. This makes them a safer option for those concerned about potential exposure to harmful substances.

- **Reduces Risk of Toxic Shock Syndrome (TSS):** While the risk of TSS is very low with any menstrual product, it's even lower with menstrual cups compared to tampons, especially when the cup is used and cleaned correctly.

5. **Comfort and Convenience**

- **Less Odor:** Because menstrual cups collect blood rather than absorbing it, and because they sit internally, they tend to produce less odor than pads and tampons.

- **Comfortable Fit:** When inserted correctly, menstrual cups can be very comfortable. Many users report that they can't feel the cup at all, allowing them to participate in all activities, including swimming and sports, without discomfort.

- **Fewer Bathroom Trips:** Since cups can hold more fluid than a tampon or pad, you don't need to worry about frequent trips to the bathroom to change your product.

6. **Holds More Fluid**

- **Capacity:** Menstrual cups can hold more fluid than tampons or pads—often between 20 to 30 milliliters (about 3 to 4 times more than a regular tampon). This makes them particularly beneficial for people with heavier flows.

7. **Good for Various Activities**

- **Active Lifestyle:** Whether you're swimming, running, hiking, or doing yoga, menstrual cups are a great option for people with active lifestyles. They stay in place securely and allow for a wide range of motion without leakage.

- **Travel-Friendly:** Because you only need one cup for your entire period, menstrual cups are convenient for travel, freeing up space in your luggage and eliminating the need to pack multiple products.

8. **Less Vaginal Dryness**

- **No Absorption of Natural Moisture:** Unlike tampons, which can absorb vaginal moisture along with menstrual blood, menstrual cups do not dry out the vagina. This helps maintain your natural pH balance and reduces the risk of irritation or discomfort.

9. **Customizable Fit**

- **Variety of Sizes:** Menstrual cups come in various sizes and shapes to fit different body types, ages, and flow levels. Some brands offer soft cups for sensitive users or firmer cups for those with stronger pelvic floor muscles, ensuring there's a cup that's right for everyone.

10. **Discreet and Low Maintenance**

- **No Need to Carry Supplies:** Once you have your menstrual cup, you don't need to carry around pads or tampons. This can be especially convenient in situations where you don't have easy access to period products.

- **Easy Maintenance:** Cleaning a menstrual cup is simple and requires just rinsing with water and soap between uses during your cycle, and boiling it at the end of your period to sanitize it.

11. **Empowerment and Body Awareness**

- **Understanding Your Body:** Using a menstrual cup can help you become more in tune with your body and your menstrual flow. It encourages you to understand your cycle better and be more comfortable with your own anatomy.

- **Less Reliance on Disposable Products:** Using a menstrual cup can be empowering, as it allows you to break free from the cycle of purchasing and disposing of single-use products.

Debunking the Myth: Do You Need to Remove a Tampon When You Pee?

This is a common misconception, but the answer is **NO, you don't need to remove a tampon when you pee**. Here's why:

The female anatomy has three separate openings: the urethra (for urine), the vagina (where the tampon is inserted), and the anus (for bowel movements). The urethra and the vaginal opening are different, which means that urine flows out of the urethra and not from the vagina. So, a tampon doesn't interfere with urination. When you pee, the tampon remains in place inside the vagina, completely unaffected by the flow of urine.

However, you might notice that the tampon string gets wet during urination. To keep it dry and clean, you can simply hold the string to the side while peeing. If it does get wet, you can gently pat it dry with toilet paper. This prevents any discomfort and helps maintain better hygiene.

Proper Care and Hygiene Tips

- **Change your tampon every 4-6 hours** to prevent bacterial growth and avoid the risk of Toxic Shock Syndrome (TSS).

- **Wash your hands** before and after inserting or removing a tampon to reduce the chance of introducing bacteria.

- If you find the tampon string irritating or it gets too wet during urination, consider switching to a pad or menstrual cup, which might be more comfortable for you.

By understanding how tampons work, you can feel more confident in using them without unnecessary concerns about urination. It's all about making informed decisions and finding the right menstrual care products that suit your body and lifestyle.

Conclusion

Menstrual cups offer numerous benefits, from cost savings and environmental protection to comfort and health advantages. They're a versatile and sustainable option for menstrual management, making them an excellent choice for many people. While there's a learning curve when you first start using a menstrual cup, the long-term benefits often outweigh the initial challenges, leading to a more convenient and eco-friendly period experience.

Menstrual cups and tampons are both popular options for managing menstruation, but they differ significantly in terms of usage, comfort, environmental impact, cost, and health considerations. Here's a detailed comparison between the two:

Both menstrual cups and tampons have their own unique benefits and drawbacks, and the best choice depends on your personal preferences, lifestyle, and comfort. Menstrual cups are more eco-friendly, cost-effective, and offer longer wear times, making them ideal for those looking for a sustainable and low-maintenance option. On the other hand, tampons are widely available, easy to use, and convenient for those who prefer a disposable option.

Ultimately, many people find that using a combination of products, such as a menstrual cup for heavy days and tampons for lighter days or specific activities, provides the best balance of comfort, convenience, and protection.

Switching to a menstrual cup can be a great decision for your health, budget, and the environment. However, there are several factors to consider to ensure a smooth transition and to find the right cup for your needs. Here's a guide to help you make the switch:

1. **Size and Fit**

- **Body Anatomy:** Menstrual cups come in different sizes, typically small and large, to accommodate different body types, age groups, and flow levels. The size you choose should be based on factors like whether you've given birth, your age, and your cervix height.

- **Small Size:** Generally recommended for those under 30 who haven't given birth vaginally.

- **Large Size:** Often suggested for those over 30 or anyone who has given birth vaginally, or those with a heavier flow.

- **Cervix Height:** Check your cervix height during your period to determine whether you need a short or long cup. A higher cervix might require a longer cup, while a lower cervix might be better suited to a shorter cup.

2. **Material Sensitivity**

- **Silicone vs. Rubber:** Most menstrual cups are made from medical-grade silicone, which is hypoallergenic and safe for most people. However, if you have a latex allergy, avoid rubber cups. Make sure to choose a material that's comfortable and safe for your body.

- **Firmness:** Some cups are firmer while others are softer. A firmer cup can open more easily but might be less comfortable for those with a sensitive bladder. A softer cup might be more comfortable but could be harder to open inside the vagina.

3. **Insertion and Removal**

- **Learning Curve:** There's often a learning curve with menstrual cups, particularly when it comes to inserting and removing the cup. It may take a few cycles to become comfortable with the process.

- **Folding Technique:** Learn different folding techniques (like the C-fold, punch-down fold, or 7-fold) to find which one works best for you.

- **Breaking the Seal:** To remove the cup, you need to break the seal by pinching the base of the cup before gently pulling it out. Practice this to avoid any discomfort.

- **Lubrication:** Using water or a water-based lubricant can help with insertion, especially when you're first getting used to the cup.

4. **Comfort**

- **Stems:** Some cups have longer stems, which can be trimmed for comfort. The stem is there to help with removal, but if it protrudes or causes discomfort, you can adjust it to your liking.

- **Positioning:** The cup should sit lower in the vaginal canal than a tampon, but you shouldn't feel it when it's in place. If you experience discomfort, try repositioning the cup or choosing a different size.

5. **Flow and Capacity**

- **Flow Level:** Consider your flow when choosing a cup. Most cups hold more fluid than a tampon, making them ideal for heavy flow days. However, if your flow is particularly heavy, you might need to empty the cup more frequently.

- **Emptying Frequency:** Depending on your flow, you may need to empty the cup every 4 to 12 hours. It's important to get used to checking the cup and knowing how often you need to empty it to avoid leaks.

6. **Maintenance and Cleaning**

- **Daily Cleaning:** After emptying the cup, rinse it with warm water and a mild, unscented soap before reinserting. Some people prefer to carry a small bottle of water or wipes for cleaning when they're on the go.

- **Sterilization:** At the end of your cycle, boil the cup in water for 5-10 minutes to sterilize it. You can also use a sterilizing solution specifically designed for menstrual cups.

- **Storage:** Store the cup in a breathable pouch (usually provided with the cup) when not in use to prevent bacterial growth.

7. **Public Bathroom Concerns**

- **Rinsing in Public:** If you need to empty your cup in a public restroom, you can wipe it clean with toilet paper or use a menstrual cup wipe.

- **Frequency of Emptying:** Because menstrual cups can hold more fluid than tampons or pads, you may not need to empty the cup as frequently, reducing the need to manage it in public restrooms.

8. **Travel and Convenience**

- **Travel-Friendly:** Menstrual cups are convenient for travel since you don't need to carry around a large supply of tampons or pads. Just ensure you have a way to clean and sterilize the cup while traveling.

- **Activity Level:** Menstrual cups are great for active lifestyles, including swimming, running, and yoga. Once properly inserted, they stay in place and provide reliable protection during physical activities.

9. **Environmental Impact**

- **Eco-Friendly Choice:** If reducing waste is a priority, a menstrual cup is one of the most eco-friendly period products available. By switching to a cup, you can significantly reduce your environmental footprint compared to using disposable products.

10. **Trial and Error**

- **Finding the Right Cup:** It might take trying out a couple of different brands or sizes before finding the one that fits best for you. Some companies offer refunds or exchanges if the cup doesn't work for you, so check the return policy before purchasing.

- **Patience and Persistence:** Don't be discouraged if you don't get it right on the first try. With a bit of practice, using a menstrual cup can become as easy and routine as using any other period product.

Conclusion

Switching to a menstrual cup can be a significant change, but it offers numerous benefits, including cost savings, environmental impact, and long-lasting comfort. By considering factors like size, material, comfort, and your lifestyle, you can find the right cup that suits your needs. Be patient with yourself as you learn to use it, and don't hesitate to seek out tips and advice from other users or the brand's customer support if needed. With time, many people find that the menstrual cup becomes their preferred period product.

Cleaning and maintaining a menstrual cup is crucial for both your health and the longevity of the cup. Proper care ensures that your cup remains safe to use, hygienic, and free from odors. Here's a step-by-step guide on how to clean and maintain your menstrual cup:

1. **Cleaning During Your Period**

Rinsing Between Uses

- **Rinse with Cold Water First:** After removing your menstrual cup, empty the contents into the toilet. Rinse the cup with cold water first to help prevent stains from setting.

- **Use Mild, Unscented Soap:** Wash the cup with warm water and a mild, unscented, oil-free soap. Make sure the soap is free from harsh chemicals, fragrances, and oils, as these can cause irritation or damage to the cup.

- **Rinse Thoroughly:** After washing, rinse the cup thoroughly with warm water to remove any soap residue, which can cause irritation or affect the cup's material.

- **Reinsert:** After cleaning, the cup is ready to be reinserted.

Cleaning in Public Restrooms

- **Wipe or Rinse with Water:** If you need to clean your cup in a public restroom, you can use menstrual cup wipes or toilet paper to wipe it clean. you can also rinse it over the toilet.

- **Carry a Backup:** Some people carry a small, clean, wet cloth or a spare cup when they know they'll be out in public for extended periods.

2. **End-of-Cycle Cleaning**

Deep Cleaning

- **Boil the Cup:** At the end of your period, it's important to sterilize your cup. Boil it in water for 5-10 minutes to kill any bacteria. Make sure the cup is fully submerged in water and that it doesn't touch the bottom of the pot, as this can cause the silicone to burn.

- **Tip:** Some people place the cup in a whisk or silicone tongs to keep it off the bottom of the pot.

- **Sterilizing Solutions:** Alternatively, you can use a sterilizing solution specifically designed for menstrual cups, or you can use sterilizing tablets (like those used for baby bottles) dissolved in water.

Removing Stains and Odors

- **Soaking in Hydrogen Peroxide:** If your cup has developed stains, you can soak it in a solution of 3% hydrogen peroxide and water (in equal parts) for a few hours. Rinse thoroughly with water afterward.

- **Baking Soda Paste:** For persistent stains, make a paste with baking soda and water, and gently scrub the cup with it. Rinse thoroughly before use.

- **Sunlight:** Letting your cup sit in direct sunlight for a few hours can naturally bleach out stains and eliminate odors.

3. **Storage Between Cycles**

- **Dry the Cup Thoroughly:** After cleaning and sterilizing, let the cup dry completely before storing it.

- **Use a Breathable Bag:** Store your cup in a breathable cotton bag (often provided by the manufacturer) or a similar breathable fabric. Avoid storing it in airtight containers, as this can encourage bacterial growth.

- **Keep in a Cool, Dry Place:** Store the cup in a cool, dry place, away from direct sunlight, which can degrade the material over time.

4. **General Maintenance Tips**

- **Inspect Regularly:** Before each use, inspect the cup for any signs of wear and tear, such as cracks, holes, or changes in texture. If the cup shows signs of damage, it's time to replace it.

- **Replace When Necessary:** With proper care, a menstrual cup can last up to 10 years. However, if you notice any significant wear or if the cup becomes sticky or discolored despite cleaning, consider replacing it sooner.

- **Avoid Harsh Cleaners:** Never use bleach, vinegar, alcohol, or oil-based soaps to clean your cup, as these can damage the silicone and cause irritation.

- **Avoid Scrubbing with Abrasive Materials:** While it's okay to use a soft cloth or brush for stubborn stains, avoid abrasive materials that could scratch the surface of the cup.

5. **Troubleshooting Common Issues**

- **Persistent Odors:** If your cup develops a persistent odor, try soaking it in a 50/50 solution of vinegar and water for an hour, followed by boiling it. Always rinse thoroughly to remove any residue.

- **Staining:** Light staining is normal and doesn't affect the performance of the cup. However, if the stains bother you, consider the cleaning tips mentioned above, like using hydrogen peroxide or sunlight exposure.

Conclusion

Proper cleaning and maintenance of your menstrual cup are essential for your health and the longevity of the cup. By following these steps, you can ensure that your cup remains clean, safe, and effective for many years. Regular cleaning during your cycle, thorough sterilization at the end of each period, and careful storage will help you get the most out of your menstrual cup while maintaining optimal hygiene.

Choosing the right tampon size is important for comfort, effectiveness, and safety during your period. Tampons come in various absorbency levels, and selecting the right one depends on your menstrual flow, personal comfort, and specific needs. Here's a guide to help you choose the right tampon size:

1. **Understand Tampon Absorbency Levels**

Tampons are categorized by their absorbency levels, which indicate how much menstrual fluid they can hold. Here's a breakdown of the common absorbency levels:

- **Light/Junior:** Suitable for light flow or the beginning and end of your period. These tampons can absorb up to 6 grams of fluid.

- **Regular/Normal:** Ideal for an average flow. These tampons absorb between 6 and 9 grams of fluid.

- **Super:** Designed for heavier flow days, absorbing between 9 and 12 grams of fluid.

- **Super Plus:** Suitable for very heavy flow, absorbing between 12 and 15 grams of fluid.

- **Ultra:** For extremely heavy flow, absorbing between 15 and 18 grams of fluid.

2. **Match the Tampon to Your Flow**

Your menstrual flow varies throughout your period, so you may need different tampon sizes on different days.

- **First and Last Days:** Your flow is typically lighter, so start with a **light/junior** or **regular/normal** tampon.

- **Heaviest Days:** During the middle of your period, when your flow is heaviest, switch to a **super** or **super plus** tampon if needed.

- **Adjust Throughout Your Period:** You might find that using a higher absorbency tampon during the day and a lower absorbency one at night works best for you.

3. **Consider Your Comfort**

Choosing the right size isn't just about absorbency; it's also about comfort.

- **Insertion:** A tampon that's too large for your flow might feel uncomfortable or difficult to insert. If you experience discomfort or difficulty inserting the tampon, try a lower absorbency option.

- **Removal:** A tampon should be easy to remove after 4-8 hours. If it feels dry or resistant when you try to remove it, it's a sign that you should use a lower absorbency tampon.

- **Comfort During Wear:** You shouldn't feel the tampon when it's properly inserted. If you do, it may not be inserted correctly, or you might need a different size.

4. **Trial and Error**

It might take some experimentation to find the right tampon size for each stage of your period.

- **Start with Regular:** If you're new to tampons or unsure of your flow, start with a **regular/normal** tampon. From there, you can adjust to a lighter or heavier absorbency depending on how well it works for you.

- **Mix and Match:** Consider using different absorbency levels on different days. For example, you might use a **super** tampon during the day and switch to **regular** at night or on lighter flow days.

5. **Consider Your Activity Level**

Your activity level can also influence your choice of tampon size.

- **Active Days:** If you're exercising or swimming, you might prefer a **super** or **super plus** tampon for added protection.

- **Less Active Days:** On days when you're less active, a **regular** or

6. **Minimize the Risk of Toxic Shock Syndrome (TSS)**

To minimize the risk of TSS, it's important to choose the lowest absorbency tampon that meets your needs.

- **Change Regularly:** Change your tampon every 4-8 hours, even if it's not fully saturated. Never leave a tampon in for more than 8 hours.

- **Use the Right Absorbency:** Avoid using a higher absorbency tampon than necessary, as this can increase the risk of TSS.

7. **Age and Experience**

Younger users or those new to tampons might prefer starting with **light/junior** tampons, which are smaller and easier to insert.

- **First-Time Users:** If it's your first time using a tampon, consider starting with a **light/junior** size to get used to the process. You can always switch to a higher absorbency as you become more comfortable.

8. **Nighttime Use**

For overnight protection, some women prefer using a **super plus** tampon. However, it's important to note that you should never leave a tampon in for more than 8 hours. If you're sleeping for longer, consider using a pad instead.

9. **Special Considerations**

- **Heavy Periods:** If you have particularly heavy periods, you might need **super** or **super plus** tampons throughout your period. However, it's still important to change tampons regularly.

- **Postpartum:** After childbirth, your flow may be heavier or different than usual. Consult with your healthcare provider about when it's safe to start using tampons again and what absorbency might be best for you.

Conclusion

Choosing the right tampon size involves understanding your menstrual flow, considering your comfort, and being mindful of safety. By selecting the appropriate absorbency level for each day of your period and adjusting as needed, you can ensure effective protection and comfort. Don't be afraid to try different sizes and brands to find what works best for you, and remember that it's normal for your needs to change over time.

10

The Fetal Position: Curl Up for Comfort

One of the most instinctive positions when dealing with period cramps is the fetal position. Curling up on your side with your knees pulled up toward your chest can help relax the muscles in your abdomen and reduce the intensity of cramps. This position is comforting because it reduces the strain on your back and abdomen, allowing your body to relax.

- **How to Do It:** Lie on your side, and bring your knees up towards your chest. You can place a pillow between your knees or under your stomach for extra support.

- **Why It Helps:** The fetal position helps to release tension in the lower back and abdominal muscles, which can relieve some of the pressure causing cramps.

The Child's Pose: A Gentle Stretch

The child's pose, a common yoga position, is another great way to relieve period cramps. This position gently stretches your back and hips, promoting relaxation and reducing pain.

- **How to Do It:** Start on your hands and knees, then lower your hips back towards your heels. Stretch your arms out in front of you, resting your forehead on the ground. Breathe deeply and hold the position for several minutes.

- **Why It Helps:** The child's pose stretches the lower back and hip muscles, which can help relieve the tension that contributes to cramps. It also encourages deep breathing, which can promote relaxation.

Legs Up the Wall: Elevation for Relief

Another simple and effective position is lying on your back with your legs elevated against a wall. This position can help improve circulation and reduce the pressure on your lower abdomen.

- **How to Do It:** Lie on your back close to a wall, then lift your legs up so they rest vertically against the wall. Keep your arms relaxed by your sides and breathe deeply.

- **Why It Helps:** Elevating your legs can help reduce swelling and improve blood flow, which may help alleviate cramp pain. It's also a very relaxing position that can help you unwind.

Pelvic Tilts: Gentle Movement

Pelvic tilts are a gentle exercise that can help relieve lower back pain and cramping. This movement helps to stretch the lower back and abdominal muscles, which can reduce tension and discomfort.

- **How to Do It:** Lie on your back with your knees bent and feet flat on the floor. Slowly tilt your pelvis upward, flattening your back against the floor. Hold for a few seconds, then release. Repeat this movement several times.

- **Why It Helps:** Pelvic tilts gently stretch and strengthen the muscles in the lower back and abdomen, which can help reduce cramping and discomfort.

Heat Therapy: Warming Up for Comfort

One of the most effective ways to relieve period cramps is through heat therapy. Applying a heating pad or hot water bottle to your lower abdomen can help relax the muscles and ease pain.

- **How to Do It:** Place a heating pad or hot water bottle on your lower abdomen, and relax in a comfortable position. Leave it in place for 15-20 minutes, or longer if needed.

- **Why It Helps:** Heat helps to increase blood flow and relax the muscles in your uterus, which can significantly reduce cramping pain.

Hydration and Nutrition: Supporting Your Body

Staying hydrated and eating a balanced diet can also play a role in reducing period cramps. Dehydration can worsen cramping, so it's important to drink plenty of water throughout the day. Additionally, certain foods can help reduce inflammation and support muscle function.

- **Stay Hydrated:** Drink plenty of water, herbal teas, or electrolyte-rich drinks. Avoid excessive caffeine and alcohol, which can contribute to dehydration.

- **Eat Anti-Inflammatory Foods:** Incorporate foods like leafy greens, berries, nuts, and fatty fish into your diet. These foods are rich in nutrients that help reduce inflammation and support overall health.

Gentle Exercise: Moving Through the Pain

While it might be the last thing you feel like doing, gentle exercise can actually help reduce period cramps. Activities like walking, yoga, or swimming can increase blood flow and release endorphins, which act as natural painkillers.

- **How to Do It:** Choose a low-impact activity that you enjoy, such as a gentle walk, a yoga session, or a swim. Focus on movements that feel good and don't push yourself too hard.

- **Why It Helps:** Exercise promotes circulation, which can reduce the severity of cramps. It also releases endorphins, which can improve your mood and reduce pain.

Breathing Techniques: Finding Calm Amidst the Pain

Deep breathing exercises can help you manage the pain of cramps by promoting relaxation and reducing stress. When you focus on your breath, it can help distract your mind from the pain and relax your muscles.

- **How to Do It:** Try diaphragmatic breathing, where you breathe deeply into your belly rather than shallow breaths into your chest. Place a hand on your abdomen, breathe in slowly through your nose, allowing your belly to rise, then exhale slowly through your mouth.

- **Why It Helps:** Deep breathing activates the parasympathetic nervous system, which promotes relaxation and can reduce the intensity of cramps.

Over-the-Counter Pain Relief: When You Need Extra Help

Sometimes, despite your best efforts, the pain can be too much to bear. In these cases, over-the-counter pain relievers like ibuprofen or naproxen can be very effective.

- **How to Use It:** Take the medication as directed on the package, ideally at the first sign of cramps. These medications work best when taken before the pain becomes too severe.

- **Why It Helps:** NSAIDs (non-steroidal anti-inflammatory drugs) like ibuprofen reduce inflammation and block the production of prostaglandins, the chemicals responsible for menstrual cramps.

Conclusion: Finding What Works for You

Period cramps can be incredibly challenging, but with the right strategies, you can find relief and comfort. Whether it's finding the perfect position to relax in, using heat therapy, or incorporating gentle exercise and breathing techniques, there are many ways to ease the pain.

Remember, every woman's body is different, and what works for one person might not work for another. It's important to try different approaches and find what provides you with the most relief. Don't hesitate to talk to your healthcare provider if your cramps are severe or if you're looking for more effective treatment options.

Ultimately, managing period cramps is about listening to your body and giving it the care and attention it needs during this time. With the right tools and techniques, you can reduce the impact of cramps on your life and continue to thrive, even on those challenging days.

This chapter provides practical advice and positions that can help alleviate period cramps, along with other strategies for pain management.

Certainly! Here are some natural remedies that can help alleviate period cramps:

1. **Heat Therapy**

- **How It Works:** Applying heat to your lower abdomen or back can relax the muscles and reduce cramping. Heat improves blood flow and can be very soothing.

- **How to Use:** Use a heating pad, hot water bottle, or take a warm bath. Apply the heat for 15-20 minutes at a time, as needed.

2. **Herbal Teas**

- **Ginger Tea:** Ginger has anti-inflammatory properties that can help reduce the production of prostaglandins, the hormones that cause cramps.

- **Chamomile Tea:** Chamomile has antispasmodic properties that can help relax the uterus and reduce cramps.

- **Peppermint Tea:** Peppermint is a natural muscle relaxant and can ease cramping and bloating.

3. **Magnesium-Rich Foods**

- **How It Works:** Magnesium helps relax muscles and can reduce the intensity of cramps. It's also known to help regulate serotonin, which can improve mood.

- **What to Eat:** Include foods like leafy green vegetables, nuts, seeds, bananas, and dark chocolate in your diet, especially leading up to and during your period.

4. **Omega-3 Fatty Acids**

- **How It Works:** Omega-3 fatty acids have anti-inflammatory properties that can reduce period pain. They help lower the production of prostaglandins, which are responsible for cramping.

- **What to Eat:** Fatty fish like salmon, mackerel, and sardines are rich in omega-3s. If you don't eat fish, consider flaxseeds, chia seeds, or an omega-3 supplement.

5. **Regular Exercise**

- **How It Works:** Exercise increases blood circulation and releases endorphins, which are natural painkillers. Regular physical activity can help reduce the severity and duration of cramps.

- **What to Do:** Engage in moderate exercise like walking, swimming, or yoga. Even gentle stretching can help relieve cramps.

6. **Essential Oils**

- **Lavender Oil:** Lavender is known for its calming properties and can help reduce pain and discomfort.

- **Clary Sage Oil:** Clary sage can balance hormones and reduce cramping.

- **Peppermint Oil:** Peppermint has cooling and muscle-relaxing effects that can soothe cramps.

- **How to Use:** Dilute essential oils with a carrier oil (like coconut or jojoba oil) and massage onto your lower abdomen. You can also add a few drops to a warm bath.

7. **Acupuncture and Acupressure**

- **How It Works:** Acupuncture involves inserting thin needles into specific points on the body to balance energy and reduce pain. Acupressure applies pressure to these points without needles.

- **What It Does:** Both techniques are thought to release endorphins and improve blood flow, which can reduce cramps.

- **How to Try:** Seek a licensed acupuncturist or try acupressure at home by pressing points like the one located three finger-widths below your navel.

8. **Hydration**

- **How It Works:** Staying hydrated helps reduce bloating, which can worsen cramps. Proper hydration also supports muscle function and can reduce the intensity of cramps.

- **What to Drink:** Drink plenty of water throughout the day. Herbal teas and electrolyte-rich drinks can also help.

9. **Calcium-Rich Foods**

- **How It Works:** Calcium helps regulate muscle contractions and can prevent the muscles in the uterus from cramping.

- **What to Eat:** Include calcium-rich foods like dairy products, fortified plant-based milk, leafy greens, almonds, and tofu in your diet.

10. **Turmeric**

- **How It Works:** Turmeric contains curcumin, an anti-inflammatory compound that can help reduce pain and inflammation associated with menstrual cramps.

- **How to Use:** Add turmeric to your meals, take it as a supplement, or make a turmeric latte with milk and honey.

11. **Vitamin D**

- **How It Works:** Vitamin D can help reduce the production of prostaglandins, which are responsible for cramping.

- **How to Get It:** Spend time in sunlight, eat vitamin D-rich foods like fatty fish and fortified foods, or take a supplement.

12. **Deep Breathing and Relaxation Techniques**

- **How It Works:** Stress can exacerbate period cramps. Deep breathing and relaxation techniques help reduce stress and promote muscle relaxation.

- **What to Do:** Practice diaphragmatic breathing, meditation, or mindfulness exercises to help manage pain.

13. **Dietary Adjustments**

- **Reduce Caffeine and Sugar:** Caffeine and sugar can increase inflammation and make cramps worse. Try reducing your intake of these during your period.

- **Eat Small, Frequent Meals:** Eating smaller meals more frequently can help maintain stable blood sugar levels and prevent cramps.

14. **Massage Therapy**

- **How It Works:** Massaging the lower abdomen with gentle pressure can help reduce tension and relieve cramps.

- **What to Do:** Use a circular motion with your fingers on your lower abdomen. You can combine this with essential oils for added relief.

15. **Sleep and Rest**

- **How It Works:** Getting enough sleep and rest can help your body recover and reduce the severity of cramps.

- **What to Do:** Aim for 7-9 hours of sleep per night and take naps if needed during your period.

Period cramps can be uncomfortable, but natural remedies offer effective ways to alleviate the pain. By combining dietary changes, gentle exercise, herbal treatments, and relaxation techniques, you can manage your cramps more effectively. Remember, it's important to listen to your body and find the combination of remedies that work best for you. If your cramps are severe or don't improve with natural treatments, it's always a good idea to consult with a healthcare professional for further advice.

Certain foods can help relieve period cramps by reducing inflammation, relaxing muscles, and providing essential nutrients that support overall menstrual health. Here are some of the best foods to incorporate into your diet to help ease cramp pain:

1. **Leafy Green Vegetables**

- **Examples:** Spinach, kale, Swiss chard, collard greens

- **Benefits:** Leafy greens are rich in magnesium, a mineral that helps relax muscles and reduce cramping. They also provide iron, which is important for replenishing blood loss during your period.

2. **Fatty Fish**

- **Examples:** Salmon, mackerel, sardines, trout

- **Benefits:** Fatty fish are high in omega-3 fatty acids, which have anti-inflammatory properties that can reduce the intensity of cramps. Omega-3s also help balance hormones and reduce prostaglandin levels, which are associated with period pain.

3. **Bananas**

- **Benefits:** Bananas are an excellent source of potassium, which helps prevent water retention and bloating. They also contain vitamin B6, which can help regulate mood and reduce irritability during your period.

4. **Nuts and Seeds**

- **Examples:** Almonds, walnuts, flaxseeds, chia seeds, pumpkin seeds

- **Benefits:** Nuts and seeds are rich in magnesium, omega-3 fatty acids, and vitamin E. Magnesium helps relax muscles, while omega-3s reduce inflammation, and vitamin E can help alleviate breast tenderness and menstrual pain.

5. **Dark Chocolate**

- **Benefits:** Dark chocolate (with at least 70% cocoa) is rich in magnesium, which helps soothe muscles and reduce cramps. It also contains antioxidants and can boost serotonin levels, improving mood during your period.

6. **Berries**
  - **Examples:** Blueberries, strawberries, raspberries, blackberries

- **Benefits:** Berries are high in antioxidants, vitamins, and fiber. Their anti-inflammatory properties can help reduce cramping, and their natural sweetness can satisfy sugar cravings without spiking blood sugar levels.

7. **Ginger**

- **Benefits:** Ginger has natural anti-inflammatory and pain-relieving properties that can help reduce the production of prostaglandins, which are responsible for cramping. It's also effective in reducing nausea that some people experience during their period.

- **How to Use:** Add fresh ginger to teas, smoothies, or meals.

8. **Turmeric**

- **Benefits:** Turmeric contains curcumin, an anti-inflammatory compound that can help alleviate period pain by reducing inflammation in the body.

- **How to Use:** Incorporate turmeric into your meals, or make a turmeric latte with warm milk and honey.

9. **Avocados**

- **Benefits:** Avocados are rich in healthy fats, potassium, magnesium, and fiber. The healthy fats help reduce inflammation, while potassium and magnesium work together to relax muscles and prevent cramping.

10. **Whole Grains**

- **Examples:** Brown rice, quinoa, oats, whole wheat

- **Benefits:** Whole grains are a good source of complex carbohydrates, which help stabilize blood sugar levels and provide sustained energy. They also contain magnesium and B vitamins, which support muscle function and reduce cramps.

11. **Watermelon and Other Hydrating Fruits**

- **Examples:** Watermelon, cucumber, oranges, melons

- **Benefits:** Staying hydrated is important during your period, as dehydration can worsen cramps. Water-rich fruits help keep you hydrated while providing vitamins and minerals that can alleviate bloating and cramps.

12. **Yogurt**

- **Benefits:** Yogurt is a good source of calcium and probiotics. Calcium helps reduce muscle spasms and cramps, while probiotics support a healthy gut, which can be beneficial for managing bloating and digestive issues during your period.

13. **Pineapple**

- **Benefits:** Pineapple contains bromelain, an enzyme with anti-inflammatory properties that can help relax muscles and reduce cramping. Pineapple is also rich in vitamin C and manganese, which support overall health.

14. **Herbal Teas**

- **Examples:** Chamomile tea, peppermint tea, ginger tea

- **Benefits:** Herbal teas, especially those with anti-inflammatory properties, can help soothe cramps and promote relaxation. Chamomile, in particular, has antispasmodic properties that can help reduce muscle cramps.

15. **Olive Oil**

- **Benefits:** Olive oil is rich in healthy monounsaturated fats and anti-inflammatory compounds. Incorporating olive oil into your diet can help reduce inflammation and support overall menstrual health.

- **How to Use:** Use olive oil in salad dressings, for cooking, or drizzling over vegetables.

Conclusion

Incorporating these nutrient-rich foods into your diet can help alleviate period cramps and support overall menstrual health. Focus on eating a balanced diet rich in anti-inflammatory foods, healthy fats, and plenty of fruits and vegetables. Staying hydrated and maintaining regular meals can also help stabilize blood sugar levels and prevent cramp-related discomfort. By making these dietary adjustments, you can help reduce the severity and duration of period cramps naturally.

Cramps, or menstrual cramps, occur as a natural part of the menstrual cycle, and they are medically known as dysmenorrhea. These cramps are caused by the contractions of the uterus as it sheds its lining. Here's a detailed explanation of why cramps occur:

1. **Role of the Uterus in Menstruation**

- **Uterine Lining (Endometrium):** Each month, the uterus prepares for a possible pregnancy by building up a thick, blood-rich lining (the endometrium). If pregnancy does not occur, this lining is no longer needed and must be shed.

- **Menstruation:** The shedding of the uterine lining is what causes menstruation, or your period. This process involves the breaking down and expelling of the endometrial tissue through the cervix and out of the body via the vagina.

Why Do Cramps Vary Among Women?

- **Individual Differences:** Every woman's body is different, which means the intensity and duration of cramps can vary widely. Factors such as genetics, hormonal levels, lifestyle, and overall health can influence the severity of menstrual cramps.

- **Age and Life Stage:** Younger women and teenagers often experience more severe cramps due to higher levels of prostaglandins. However, cramps may lessen with age or after childbirth as hormonal balance shifts.

7. **Managing and Reducing Cramps**

While cramps are a normal part of the menstrual cycle for many women, they can be managed and reduced through various methods:

- **Hormonal Birth Control:** Birth control pills, patches, or IUDs can regulate or reduce menstruation, leading to fewer or less intense cramps.

- **Lifestyle Changes:** Regular exercise, a healthy diet, and stress management can also help reduce the severity of cramps.

- **Heat Therapy:** Applying a heating pad to the lower abdomen can relax the uterine muscles and ease pain.

Conclusion

Menstrual cramps occur due to the natural process of the uterus contracting to shed its lining during menstruation. The intensity of these cramps can vary depending on factors like prostaglandin levels, flow intensity, and individual health. While cramps are a common experience, understanding the underlying causes can help in finding effective ways to manage and reduce the pain. If cramps are severe or interfere significantly with daily life, it's always a good idea to consult with a healthcare provider for further evaluation and management options.

11

PCOS - We Bloat, We Look for Snacks, No One Understands, and They Think We Are Lazy**

Introduction:

Meet Anisha, a woman who has been dealing with Polycystic Ovary Syndrome (PCOS) for years. PCOS is more than just a medical condition for Anisha; it's a lifestyle, and not by choice. From the endless search for snacks to the constant battle with bloating, Anisha's journey is full of challenges and humor that anyone with PCOS can relate to.

Part 1: The Uninvited Bloat

Anisha wakes up one morning feeling like a balloon that's about to burst. "Did I eat a truckload of sodium last night?" she wonders as she stares at her swollen belly in the mirror. This bloating is different from the usual post-pizza puffiness; it's the dreaded PCOS bloat that makes her feel like she's been inflated with a bicycle pump. The worst part? Explaining this to people who don't understand.

Part 2: The Snack Monster

Cravings are a normal part of life, but for Anisha, they're

like a tidal wave of hunger that strikes out of nowhere. One minute, she's content, and the next, she's scouring the kitchen for something, anything, to satisfy her insatiable hunger. She jokes that PCOS is like having a snack monster living inside her, demanding offerings at all hours of the day.

Part 3: The "Lazy" Label

Despite her best efforts, Anisha often feels misunderstood. Friends and coworkers think she's lazy when she cancels plans or takes a day off work. They don't see the fatigue that comes with PCOS or the mental exhaustion of dealing with symptoms that seem never-ending. Anisha laughs it off, but deep down, it's frustrating. "If only they knew what a day in my life was really like," she thinks, reaching for another snack.

Part 4: Humor as a Shield

To cope with the challenges, Anisha uses humor as her shield. She jokes about her "food baby" and refers to her bloated days as "pregnant with a burrito." It's her way of taking control, of not letting PCOS define her. But even in her humor, there's a hint of sadness, a wish that she didn't have to explain herself so often.

12

Planning early periods by eating pappaiya or hot items

I Invited My Period on Sunday, but It Came on Friday and Next Month It Didn't Show Up**

Should u plan your period ???

Periods are a natural part of life, but many of us are left wondering if there's any way to plan or manage them better, especially when we have important events coming up. While we can't control the exact timing of our period without medical intervention, we can certainly manage the symptoms, reduce discomfort, and even prepare our body to have a smoother menstrual cycle by being mindful of our lifestyle and diet. This chapter dives into practical tips, myth-busting advice, and the power of nutrition in planning your period.

Understanding Your Menstrual Cycle

The first step in planning your period is understanding your own cycle. A typical menstrual cycle lasts anywhere between 21 to 35 days, with periods themselves lasting for 3 to 7 days. Keeping track of your cycle using a period tracker or app can help you anticipate when your period is likely to start. With this information, you can plan important events like vacations, social gatherings, or exams around your cycle. While it's not foolproof, being aware of your cycle helps you stay prepared.

Myth-Busting: Does Papaya Really Induce Periods?

One of the most popular myths you might have heard is that eating papaya can induce your period or help it arrive sooner. The truth is, while certain foods like raw papaya are believed to stimulate uterine contractions due to the presence of an enzyme called **papain**, there's no scientific evidence to support the idea that it can actually alter your cycle or induce your period. However, papaya can help regulate menstrual flow by supporting the health of the uterus and overall hormonal balance. So, you can safely enjoy papaya as part of your diet without worrying about drastic changes to your cycle.

Other commonly suggested foods like pineapple, sesame seeds, or jaggery are also considered beneficial for period regulation due to their heat-producing properties, but they won't magically bring on a period or delay it.

Diet and Lifestyle for a Healthier Cycle

Even though foods can't manipulate your cycle directly, a balanced diet plays a crucial role in maintaining a healthy period. Here's what you can do:

1. **Eat Iron-Rich Foods:** Since periods cause blood loss, consuming iron-rich foods like spinach, lentils, and lean meats helps replenish your body's iron levels, reducing the risk of anemia.

2. **Include Healthy Fats:** Omega-3 fatty acids found in fish, chia seeds, and walnuts can help reduce inflammation and manage menstrual cramps.

3. **Hydration is Key:** Staying hydrated is crucial for minimizing bloating and preventing dehydration, which can

worsen cramps.

4. **Cut Down on Caffeine and Sugar:** Both caffeine and sugary foods can exacerbate PMS symptoms and lead to mood swings.

5. **Exercise Regularly:** Light exercise, like walking or yoga, can alleviate cramps and improve your mood, making the period days more bearable.

Preparing for Events and Special Occasions

If you have a big event or vacation planned, and your period is due around the same time, don't panic! While you can't control the exact date, here are some tips to minimize discomfort and navigate the days more comfortably:

- **Consult Your Doctor:** If you absolutely need to postpone or prepone your period for a special reason, consult your gynecologist. They might prescribe hormonal pills, but it's important to remember this option should be used sparingly and only under medical supervision.

- **Prepare a Period Kit:** Carry a small pouch with tampons, pads, or menstrual cups, along with painkillers, wet wipes, and an extra pair of underwear. Being prepared helps reduce stress and ensures that an unexpected start doesn't ruin your plans.

- **Plan Your Wardrobe:** Wear comfortable, darker clothing and consider using double protection, like a tampon and a pad, to prevent any leaks or embarrassment during social events. ### Final Thoughts: Embrace and Prepare

Planning your period is not just about timing—it's about understanding your body, embracing the changes, and finding ways to reduce discomfort so that your menstrual cycle becomes a part of your life, not an interruption. Remember, every woman's body is unique, and it's okay to have different experiences. With a little preparation and self-care, you can navigate through any period day with confidence and grace.

13

Why Are Women Stopped from Visiting Temples During Periods?

Throughout history, menstruation has been a subject of many myths, taboos, and restrictions, particularly when it comes to religious practices. One of the most debated topics is the restriction on women visiting temples during their periods. This belief is deeply ingrained in many cultures, especially in South Asia, and has led to generations of women being excluded from participating in religious rituals and ceremonies.

In this chapter, we will explore the historical, cultural, and religious reasons behind this practice and how the perception of menstruation is changing in modern times.

The Concept of Purity and Impurity

The primary reason behind this restriction is the concept of ritual purity and impurity. In many traditional beliefs, menstruation is considered a state of "impurity" or "pollution." This notion comes from the idea that anything associated with blood, bodily fluids, or internal processes was not well understood in ancient times and was therefore seen as something that should be kept away from sacred spaces.

This idea of impurity is not limited to menstruation. Many cultures also have restrictions on people who are dealing with other bodily changes, like post-childbirth recovery or certain health conditions. Such restrictions are part of broader rituals aimed at maintaining the "purity" of sacred spaces.

Hygiene and Health Concerns in the Past

In the past, when there was limited understanding of the menstrual cycle and lack of access to proper hygiene products, women faced difficulties in managing their periods. They didn't have access to the sanitary napkins, tampons, or menstrual cups we have today. During those times, restricting women from visiting temples or participating in public activities may have been a way to ensure rest and hygiene.

Also female were stopped going at temple because earlier temple were located at mountain and during periods female need rest so it was decided to avoid travelling or climbing mountain women were asked to take rest. But meaning of giving rest to female is taken in a different ways.

Cultural Norms and Patriarchy

Like many other restrictions imposed on women, the practice of preventing menstruating women from entering temples is also rooted in patriarchal norms. It became a way to control women's bodies and restrict their participation in social and religious life. By defining menstruation as something shameful or impure, society was able to limit women's roles and freedom.

The stigma and taboo associated with menstruation have been perpetuated by these beliefs, leading to generations of women feeling ashamed or embarrassed during their periods. This control over women's bodily functions contributed to reinforcing the idea that women are somehow lesser or unworthy during this natural process.

Spiritual Beliefs and Energy

There is also a spiritual explanation for these restrictions. Some believe that menstruation is a period when a woman's energy is at a heightened state. According to these beliefs, this energy might interfere with the spiritual vibrations of a temple. Therefore, women were asked to stay away to avoid disrupting the energy of the sacred space.

Another interpretation is that menstruating women have a higher "spiritual energy" that needs to be conserved and protected. This led to the belief that their energy should not be exposed in ritual spaces, as it might disrupt the existing balance.

Respect for Rest and Rejuvenation

In some communities, the restriction on temple visits is seen as a way of respecting a woman's need for rest and rejuvenation during her periods. By not participating in household chores or religious activities, women were traditionally given a break from their regular duties. While this might seem considerate, it is still based on the underlying belief that menstruation makes a woman less capable or pure.

Regional and Cultural Variations

Interestingly, not all temples enforce this rule. While some temples have strict restrictions, others celebrate menstruation as a sign of fertility and life. For instance, the Kamakhya Temple in Assam celebrates the annual menstruation of the goddess during the Ambubachi Mela. In this temple, menstruation is considered a symbol of the creative power of the feminine and is revered rather than shunned.

This shows that the perception of menstruation varies greatly, even within the same cultural and religious contexts.

Changing Perspectives in Modern Times

With increased awareness and education, many people today are questioning the relevance of such restrictions. Women's rights activists, religious reformists, and even some temple authorities are advocating for removing these taboos. The focus is shifting towards considering menstruation as a natural process that should not prevent a woman from participating in any activity.

In recent years, there have been several court cases and public debates in countries like India to lift these restrictions, especially in places like the **Sabarimala Temple**. Many women are now asserting their right to worship and participate in religious activities, regardless of their menstrual status.

Key Issues Covered In Sabrimala Case

1. Does the prohibition on menstruating women's entry in the Sabarimala Temple violate the Right to Equality and the Right against discrimination and the abolition of untouchability?
2. Are Lord Ayyappa's devotees a separate religious denomination, hence bearing the right to manage the administration of their own affairs in matters of religion?
3. Is women's exclusion an 'essential religious practice' under Article 25?
4. Does Rule 3 of Kerala Hindu Places of Public Worship (Authorisation of Entry) Rules permit a 'religious denomination' to ban the entry of women between the ages of 10 and 50 years.
5. Do the Public Worship Rules allowing the custom go against the parent legislation, which disallowed discriminatory practices?

The exclusion of women was first challenged at the Kerala High Court. In 1991, the Kerala High Court in S. Mahendran v The Secretary, Travancore held that the exclusion was constitutional and justified, as it was a long-standing custom. The practice did not violate women devotees' Rights to Equality and Freedom of worship.

The State of Kerala initially supported the exclusion but changed their stance mid-way. They submitted that women should be allowed entry into the temple, as age based restriction (between ages 10-50) on women can turn out to be a lifelong restriction—there is no guarantee that women would live as long as 50-55 years. They argued that customary practices can be struck down by the court for fundamental rights violation.

Sabarimala Case Conclusion

The Sabarimala temple case was a landmark ruling in India that redefined the discourse around gender equality, religious freedoms, and constitutional rights. In 2018, the Supreme Court of India delivered a 4:1 majority verdict, lifting the ban that prevented women of menstruating age (10-50 years) from entering the temple. The court held that the practice of exclusion violated the right to equality and freedom of religion, emphasizing that notions of purity and impurity related to menstruation cannot be considered essential religious practices. This judgment was seen as a victory for women's rights and equality, yet it sparked widespread debate and protests, with a significant section of devotees opposing the decision as an infringement on religious customs.

In the aftermath, the case has continued to evolve. In 2019, the Supreme Court referred the matter to a larger constitutional bench, acknowledging the complex interplay between faith, tradition, and gender equality. While the verdict technically permits entry for women of all ages, the situation on the ground remains contentious, with the temple witnessing resistance to the implementation of the order. The Sabarimala case remains a potent reminder of the ongoing tension between tradition and modernity, as well as the broader struggle for gender justice within deeply entrenched cultural and religious contexts in India.

Conclusion

The restriction on visiting temples during menstruation is primarily based on a combination of historical, cultural, and spiritual beliefs that are now being questioned and challenged. It is a reflection of how society has viewed women's bodies for centuries, often with misunderstanding and unnecessary stigma.

Today, as we become more aware and educated, it's time to change this narrative. Menstruation is not something that should hold women back from experiencing the divine or participating in any ritual. It's a natural biological process, a symbol of life and creation. It's time to move beyond these outdated practices and allow every woman to feel empowered, no matter what time of the month it is.

As we rethink these age-old beliefs, let's advocate for a more inclusive and equal society where no woman feels unworthy or impure because of a natural process. The power to redefine these norms starts with understanding, empathy, and a willingness to change.

14

Appeal – Embracing Period Leave: A Step Towards Corporate Equality

The Need for Period Leave in the Corporate World

Periods are a natural physiological process, yet they continue to be shrouded in silence and stigma, especially in the workplace. The concept of period leave has sparked debates worldwide—some argue it's a step towards gender equality, while others view it as unnecessary. The reality is that menstruation is not just a routine occurrence for many women; it often comes with debilitating pain, cramps, fatigue, and emotional fluctuations that can impact productivity and overall well-being. While women have historically been expected to power through these symptoms, there is a growing recognition of the need for compassionate policies in the corporate world, including paid period leave.

Implementing period leave doesn't suggest that women are less capable or weaker. Instead, it acknowledges the unique health challenges faced by half the workforce. By offering a one day off each month, companies can foster a more inclusive and supportive environment, ultimately boosting employee morale and retention. While some countries like Japan, South Korea, and Indonesia have enacted menstrual leave policies, the global corporate landscape still has a long way to go. It's time we shifted the narrative from viewing periods as a taboo to embracing policies that recognize and respect women's health needs.

Real-Life Case Study: Zomato's Menstrual Leave Policy

A pioneering example in India is Zomato, one of the leading food delivery companies, which introduced period leave for its female and transgender employees in 2020. This move was met with a mixture of praise and criticism. While some saw it as a progressive step towards employee welfare, others felt it might reinforce gender bias. However, the decision-makers at Zomato were clear in their vision: to create an inclusive workplace that values every employee's health and well-being.

Through their policy, Zomato offers up to 10 days of period leave annually, encouraging women and transgender employees to take a break if they need it without fear of judgment or stigma. Many employees reported feeling relieved and validated by this policy, as they no longer had to justify their discomfort or push through painful symptoms in silence. One employee shared her experience: "There were days when I'd sit in front of my screen, unable to concentrate because of severe cramps. With period leave, I no longer feel pressured to hide my pain or pretend to be okay when I'm not." Zomato's policy has not only sparked discussions on period leave in India but also paved the way for other companies to reevaluate their stance on menstrual health and employee well-being.

A Global Appeal: It's Time to Embrace Menstrual Leave

The introduction of period leave policies should not be seen as a privilege but as a fundamental health right. Women make up a significant portion of the global workforce, and it's essential to ensure that their health is prioritized. Period leave can reduce absenteeism, foster greater productivity in the long run, and create a culture of empathy and understanding. Implementing such policies globally could also break down the stigma around menstruation, encouraging open conversations about menstrual health in the workplace.

To the leaders and decision-makers of the corporate world, it's time to act. We urge companies to explore, understand, and implement period leave policies that suit their organizational structure and workforce needs. It's not just about offering a day off; it's about recognizing that women's health should never be a barrier to their professional growth. By embracing menstrual leave, we can set a new standard of equality and compassion, ensuring that women don't have to choose between their health and their career.

Thanks Note

A heartfelt thanks to the pioneers who have already taken the brave step towards introducing period leave in their organizations. Your courage and empathy inspire others to create a more inclusive and supportive corporate environment. To those still on the fence, remember that a small step today can lead to a giant leap in creating a balanced and equitable world for future generations. Let's break the cycle of stigma and foster workplaces where every individual's health is valued and respected. Together, we can shape a world that not only talks about change but also implements it.

15

Sanitary Pad Disposal in Corporate Offices—Creating a Hygienic and Inclusive Workspace

Corporate offices around the world are increasingly adopting innovative solutions to manage menstrual waste effectively, ensuring a safe and hygienic environment for all employees. Among these solutions is the installation of **Sanitary Pad Disposal Machines** in women's restrooms. These machines are designed to provide a private and convenient way for women to dispose of used pads while promoting cleanliness and proper waste management. Yet, introducing these facilities is just one part of the solution; the real impact comes from educating employees, particularly new joiners, on using these machines correctly.

Educating New Employees: A Vital Step for Success

For many new female employees, especially those accustomed to traditional disposal methods, encountering these machines for the first time can be confusing. At home, it might be common to wrap up used pads and toss them in the dustbin, but this approach can cause significant issues in an office setting. Improper disposal can lead to clogged toilets, unpleasant odors, and an unhygienic environment, which not only affects restroom conditions but also creates additional work for housekeeping staff.

This is why education and awareness are critical. Corporates must integrate sanitary pad disposal information into their onboarding process. HR teams should include this as part of the orientation program, highlighting how to use these machines properly, and explaining why they are necessary for maintaining a clean and healthy workspace.

How the Sanitary Pad Disposal Machine Works

The disposal machines are user-friendly and designed to ensure privacy. Here's a quick breakdown of how they function:
   1. **Placing the Pad**: Employees place their wrapped sanitary pad in the designated slot.
   2. **Activation**: Depending on the machine's model, it may require pressing a button or may be automatically activated by a sensor.
   3. **Shredding or Compacting**: The machine shreds or compacts the pad, sealing it in an odor-controlled compartment.
   4. **Collection and Disposal**: The waste is collected regularly and sent to appropriate facilities, where it is either incinerated or disposed of safely to prevent environmental harm.
   Advanced machines even have incineration capabilities, converting pads into non-toxic ash on the spot. This method eliminates the risk of contamination and reduces waste volume significantly.

Ensuring Proper Waste Management and Disposal

Once the pads are collected, they are typically sent to certified waste management facilities where they undergo safe disposal processes, such as incineration. If the pads are biodegradable, they may be directed to composting facilities, though this is rare due to the synthetic materials in most pads. Proper management not only ensures hygiene but also reflects a company's commitment to environmental responsibility.

Creating Awareness and Shared Responsibility

To make these machines truly effective, companies need to foster a culture of awareness and shared responsibility. This can be achieved through:

- **Visual Guides**: Clear signages and posters inside restrooms to guide employees on correct usage.

- **Workshops and Sessions**: Regular educational sessions on menstrual health and hygiene.

- **Digital Resources**: Short videos or digital guides provided during onboarding or via email.

- **Feedback Mechanisms**: Channels for employees to report any issues or share suggestions.

Final Thoughts: A Step Towards Better Hygiene and Comfort

Implementing sanitary pad disposal machines in corporate offices is not just about hygiene; it's about creating a supportive environment where women feel respected and valued. Companies that invest in these solutions, along with educational initiatives, demonstrate a genuine commitment to employee well-being and gender inclusivity. As we continue to break the stigma around menstruation, it's time for every organization to step up and provide the facilities and awareness needed to ensure a clean, safe, and comfortable workspace for all.

Thank You

We extend our gratitude to all organizations that are leading the way in promoting menstrual hygiene management. Your efforts not only contribute to a healthier work environment but also set a precedent for others to follow. Let's continue to raise awareness, support our female employees, and create workplaces where everyone can thrive comfortably and confidently.

Hope you enjoyed reading 7 Shades of Red !!.
Well now it's time to know about me

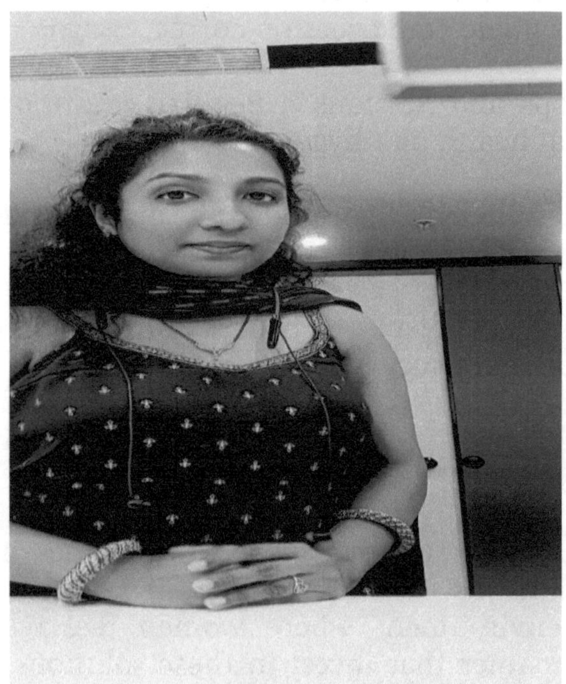

This is Hanisha Varma, I am working professional, Author, Youtuber. This is my second time attempt to connect to people, touch people heart by writing down my thoughts on female mind.

Well, I leave this up to my readers whether they felt connected or not!!

But with this book I have tried to put my thoughts in words and if I am able to change the mindset of even one person then I will feel like my mission is accomplished.

There is something more I do in my life to change the world.

I have my youtube channel in the name of Corporate Saheli Hany&Tech.

In this channel I cover Ms Office, Cyberfraud Prevention, Banking tech knowledge, Powerbi, Tableau related videos from Basic to advance tips and much more about the Digital World.

You can watch now and hit the the subscribe button if you like my contents

Those who wants to search me on youtube, Instagram simply type Hanisha Varma or Corporatesaheli Hany&Tech

Stay connected, World is yours!!

Written By Hanisha Varma

Email id – hanyandtech2021@gmail.com